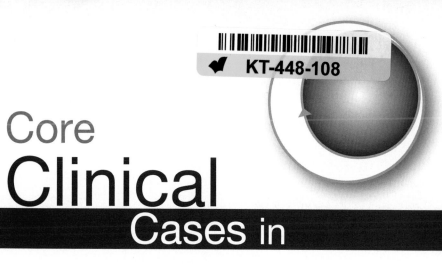

Core
Clinical
Cases in

Surgery
and Surgical
Specialties

Second edition

Edited by

Janesh K Gupta MSc MD FRCOG
Professor in Obstetrics and Gynaecology, University
of Birmingham, Birmingham Women's Hospital,
Birmingham, UK

Janesh K Gupta is also the Editor of the Core Clinical
Cases Series.

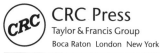

CRC Press
Taylor & Francis Group
Boca Raton London New York

CRC Press is an imprint of the
Taylor & Francis Group, an **informa** business

CRC Press
Taylor & Francis Group
6000 Broken Sound Parkway NW, Suite 300
Boca Raton, FL 33487-2742

© 2015 by Taylor & Francis Group, LLC
CRC Press is an imprint of Taylor & Francis Group, an Informa business

No claim to original U.S. Government works

Printed on acid-free paper
Version Date: 20140818

International Standard Book Number-13: 978-1-4441-7996-5 (Paperback)

This book contains information obtained from authentic and highly regarded sources. While all reasonable efforts have been made to publish reliable data and information, neither the author[s] nor the publisher can accept any legal responsibility or liability for any errors or omissions that may be made. The publishers wish to make clear that any views or opinions expressed in this book by individual editors, authors or contributors are personal to them and do not necessarily reflect the views/opinions of the publishers. The information or guidance contained in this book is intended for use by medical, scientific or health-care professionals and is provided strictly as a supplement to the medical or other professional's own judgement, their knowledge of the patient's medical history, relevant manufacturer's instructions and the appropriate best practice guidelines. Because of the rapid advances in medical science, any information or advice on dosages, procedures or diagnoses should be independently verified. The reader is strongly urged to consult the relevant national drug formulary and the drug companies' printed instructions, and their websites, before administering any of the drugs recommended in this book. This book does not indicate whether a particular treatment is appropriate or suitable for a particular individual. Ultimately it is the sole responsibility of the medical professional to make his or her own professional judgements, so as to advise and treat patients appropriately. The authors and publishers have also attempted to trace the copyright holders of all material reproduced in this publication and apologize to copyright holders if permission to publish in this form has not been obtained. If any copyright material has not been acknowledged please write and let us know so we may rectify in any future reprint.

Library of Congress Cataloging-in-Publication Data

Core clinical cases in surgery and surgical specialties / editor, Janesh K. Gupta. -- Second edition.
  p. ; cm.
  Includes bibliographical references and index.
  ISBN 978-1-4441-7996-5 (hardcover : alk. paper)
  I. Gupta, Janesh Kumar, editor.
  [DNLM: 1. Surgical Procedures, Operative--Case Reports. 2. Surgical Procedures, Operative--Problems and Exercises. 3. General Surgery--Case Reports. 4. General Surgery--Problems and Exercises. WO 18.2]

  RD37.2
  617.0076--dc23   2014028481

**Visit the Taylor & Francis Web site at
http://www.taylorandfrancis.com**

**and the CRC Press Web site at
http://www.crcpress.com**

Contents

Contributors

Nicole Abdul MBChB, BMedSci
Academic Clinical Fellow, Year 2 in Trauma and Orthopaedic Surgery,
Health Education North East, England

Matthew Clark BHB MBChB MD FRACS
Associate Professor of Surgery, University of Auckland, Middlemore Hospital,
Counties Manukau District Health Board, Auckland, New Zealand

Chris Coulson PhD FRCS
Queen Elizabeth Hospitals, Birmingham, United Kingdom

Adrian Drake-Lee MMedEd PhD FRCS
Honorary Clinical Senior Lecturer, The School of Clinical and Experimental Medicine,
The Medical School, University of Birmingham, Edgbaston, Birmingham

Suresh Ganta M Phil FRCS Urol
Consultant Urological Surgeon, Manor Hospital, Walsall, West Midlands, United Kingdom

Terence McLoughlin BSc (hon) MBChB
Emergency Medicine Specialist, NHS Mersey Deanery, United Kingdom

Desirée Murray FRCOphth
The University of the West Indies, Department of Clinical Surgical Sciences,
Eric Williams Medical Sciences Complex, Mount Hope, Trinidad and Tobago, West Indies

Jevan Taylor MBBS FRCS (GenSurg)
Consultant Oncoplastic and Reconstructive Breast Surgeon, Worcestershire Acute NHS Trust,
Worcestershire, England

Steven Thrush FRCS (GenSurg)
Consultant Breast and General Surgeon, Senior Lecturer, University of Worcester,
Worcestershire, United Kingdom

Abbreviations

A&E	accident and emergency
AAA	abdominal aortic aneurysm
ABG	arterial blood gas
ABPIs	ankle brachial pressure indices
AMD	age-related macular degeneration
ALT	alanine aminotransaminase
AREDS	Age-Related Eye Disease Study
AST	aspartate aminotransaminase
ATLS	Advanced Trauma Life Support
AUR	acute urinary retention
BCR	bulbocavernosus reflex
BIPP	bismuth iodoform paraffin paste
BP	blood pressure
BPH	benign prostatic hyperplasia
BPPV	benign positional paroxysmal vertigo
CBD	common bile duct
CSF	cerebrospinal fluid
CT	computed tomography
CTA	CT angiography
CUR	chronic urinary retention
CVA	cerebrovascular accident
DCIS	ductal carcinoma in situ
DCR	dacryocystorhinostomy
DRE	digital rectal examination
DSA	digital subtraction angiography
EBV	Epstein Barr virus
ERCP	endoscopic retrograde cholangiopancreatography
ESR	erythrocyte sedimentation rate
ESWL	extracorporeal shock wave lithotripsy
FFP	fresh frozen plasma
FISH	fluorescence in situ hybridization
FNAC	fine-needle aspiration cytology

GP	general practitioner
Hb	haemoglobin
HNPCC	hereditary non-polyposis colorectal cancer
HoLEP	holmium laser enucleation of prostate
HRCT	high-resolution computed tomography
IC	intermittent claudication
ICA	internal carotid artery
ICP	increased intracranial pressure
IOL	intraocular lens
IVU	intravenous urogram
LFT	liver function test
MCA	middle cerebral artery
MRCP	magnetic resonance cholangiopancreatography
MRI	magnetic resonance imaging
MSU	midstream urine
NSAID	non-steroidal anti-inflammatory drug
Nd:YAG	neodymium:yttrium-aluminium-garnet laser
PCA	posterior communicating artery
PCNL	percutaneous nephrolithotomy
PCPT	prostate cancer prevention trial
PCV	packed cell volume
PSA	prostate-specific antigen
PUJ	pelviureteric junction
PUK	peripheral ulcerative keratitis
PV	plasma viscosity
PVD	peripheral vascular disease
PVD	posterior vitreous detachment
RAPD	relative afferent pupillary defect
RD	retinal detachment
RP	retinitis pigmentosa
SBO	small bowel obstruction
SLE	systemic lupus erythematosus
SLN	sentinel lymph node
SUFE	slipped upper femoral epiphysis
TCC	transitional cell carcinoma

TED	thromboembolic deterrent stocking
TED	thyroid eye disease (Chap. 3)
TIA	transient ischemic attack
TNM	tumours, node, metastases
TRUS	trans-rectal ultrasound of the prostate
TURBT	trans-urethral resection of the bladder tumour
TURP	trans-urethral resection of the prostate
U&Es	urea and electrolytes
USI	urodynamic stress incontinence
UTI	urinary tract infection
VEGF	vascular endothelial growth factor
XGPN	xanthogranulomatous pyelonephritis
WCC	white cell count

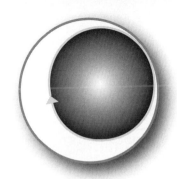

1 General surgery

Matthew Clark, Jevan Taylor, Steven Thrush

KEY CONCEPTS

HERNIAS

GALLSTONES

APPENDICITIS

COLON AND RECTAL CANCER

SURGICAL EMERGENCIES

VASCULAR: ABDOMINAL AORTIC ANEURYSM

KEY CONCEPTS

Complications can occur early or late in the post-operative period, and can be specific to the surgery performed, or more general, occurring after almost all operations.

Landmarks for post-operative care and complications

FIRST 24 HOURS

Primary haemorrhage is the most common feature presenting as tachycardia. Initially a fit young patient will have a stable blood pressure (BP) because the cardiovascular system is able to compensate. As circulating volume falls further (>20–40 per cent), hypotension develops. Resuscitation with colloid plus blood and stopping the haemorrhage is essential before decompensation occurs.

A raised temperature (<37.9°C) in the first 24-hour period is usually a reactive post-operative pyrexia, but a rise >38°C is suspicious of a urinary tract infection (UTI) that was pre-existing but flared up after urinary catheterization.

24 TO 72 HOURS

Infection of the urinary tract, chest, surgical wounds and legs (deep vein thrombosis) must be checked for causes of pyrexia during this time period.

After abdominal surgery, a pyrexia in this time period should also raise suspicion of direct injury to the bowel that was missed during surgery and has caused peritonitis.

7 TO 10 DAYS

- Secondary haemorrhage caused by infection
- Thrombosis (deep vein thrombosis or pulmonary embolus)
- Bowel anastomotic leak
- Infected post-operative collection
- Fistula formation from avascular necrosis (diathermy burns) presenting as late complications (e.g. ureteric fistula, vesicovaginal fistula, rectovaginal fistula or bowel perforation causing peritonitis)
- Pressure sores

Late complications of surgery

- Incisional hernia
- Adhesions
- False aneurysm
- Infected prosthesis

The five Bs

Who needs emergency out-of-hours surgery? Remember the five 'B's:

Block (e.g. bowel obstruction)
Bleed (e.g. peptic ulcer)
Burst (e.g. ectopic pregnancy, perforated bowel)
Break (e.g. open fractures)
Burn (e.g. skin burns)

HERNIAS

Questions

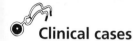
Clinical cases

For each of the clinical case scenarios given

Q1: What is the likely differential diagnosis?
Q2: What features of the given history support the diagnosis?
Q3: What additional features in the history would you seek to support a particular diagnosis?
Q4: What clinical examination would you perform and why?
Q5: What investigations would be most useful and why?
Q6: What treatment options are appropriate?

CASE 1.1 – 'I've developed a lump in my groin'

A 25-year-old builder suddenly develops a golf-ball-sized, slightly tender lump in his right groin after lifting a 20-kg bag of sand. He states that he felt a tearing sensation as it happened. He attends the accident and emergency department.

CASE 1.2 – 'I can't push my lump back in anymore'

A 70-year-old retired man presents to surgical outpatient clinic with a slightly tender lump in his left groin. He has had the lump for many months, but previously it would disappear overnight, or if necessary he could gently push it back inside. His health is fine, other than a cough from years of smoking. Over the last 2 weeks he has not been able to reduce the lump.

CASE 1.3 – 'My hernia is sore and I've started to vomit'

A slim 73-year-old woman has had a groin lump for some time which she ignored. Over the last 3 days it has become progressively more painful, with redness of the overlying skin. She has not opened her bowels during this time (which is unusual for her), and yesterday she started to vomit.

👥 OSCE Counselling cases

OSCE COUNSELLING CASE 1.1 – 'Should I have my hernia repaired?'

A 47-year-old man presents, via his general practitioner (GP), with an intermittent left groin mass, causing only moderate symptoms. Examination confirms an easily reducible inguinal hernia.

Q1: If an operation is offered, what specific risks should the patient be warned about?

OSCE COUNSELLING CASE 1.2 – 'Why did my surgeon suggest I see a urologist first?'

An otherwise well 74-year-old man has a right inguinal hernia and chooses to proceed with hernia repair. In his history he reveals that he has slight difficulty initiating urination, poor stream and nocturia. The surgeon suggests that he is seen by a urologist before proceeding with the operation.

Q1: What factors might the surgeon be thinking about in deferring the operation?
Q2: What will the urologist do?

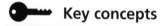 **Key concepts**

In order to work through the core clinical cases in this section you will need to understand the following key concepts.

WHAT IS A HERNIA?

'An abnormal protrusion of a viscus through the wall of the cavity that usually contains it.'

WHERE DO THEY OCCUR?

Hernias may occur anywhere in the body. Groin hernias are the most common, usually occurring through the inguinal or femoral canals. Other sites for hernias are where musculofascial weaknesses may develop (umbilicus, diaphragm, edge of rectus abdominis, lumbar triangle), when abnormally raised pressure develops (cerebral tumours causing 'coning') or as a complication of wound healing (incisional hernias).

WHAT CAN THEY CONTAIN?

Just about anything. Omentum and small bowel are the most common contents of abdominal wall hernias, but most organs (including the pregnant uterus) have been described in hernias. Sometimes the organ within the hernia sac may be pathological, such as Meckel's diverticulum (the rare Littre's hernia).

WHY ARE THEY IMPORTANT?

As well as pain from the hernia itself, their main importance relates to the complications arising from their contents. Fibrosis may lead to irreducibility of the contents (incarceration) and possibly obstruction of any contained bowel. If the blood supply of the contents is compromised, this may cause ischaemia (strangulation), necrosis and even perforation.

Answers

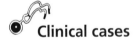

Clinical cases

CASE 1.1 – 'I've developed a lump in my groin'

A1: What is the likely differential diagnosis?

- Inguinal hernia
- Femoral hernia
- Enlarged inguinal lymph node
- Lipoma
- Less likely: groin abscess, undescended testis, saphena varix, femoral artery aneurysm, psoas abscess, tumour

A2: What features of the given history support the diagnosis?

Groin hernias may be caused by heavy exertion, but often this is not the case and no precipitating event is reported. Tenderness is common, particularly in an acute onset hernia, but may also be a feature of an enlarged lymph node or psoas abscess (signs of systemic illness would also be expected). The patient's young age makes the rarer conditions less likely.

A3: What additional features in the history would you seek to support a particular diagnosis?

Ask whether the patient has had a hernia before (making future hernias more likely) and about a family history of hernias. Does he inject into his groin? Has he been otherwise well?

A4: What clinical examination would you perform and why?

Examine the groins and external genitalia. The features characteristic of an uncomplicated hernia are a cough impulse and reducibility. An inguinal hernia passing through the deep inguinal ring is called 'indirect', and one passing through the medial posterior wall of the inguinal canal is called 'direct'. Distinguishing between the two types is possible, but makes no difference to treatment.

A5: What investigations would be most useful and why?

- Ultrasound to possibly define clinically unclear entities
- Fine-needle aspiration cytology (FNAC) of enlarged lymph nodes

A6: What treatment options are appropriate?

- Supportive: hernia trusses have been used in the past but have no role now.
- Medical: no role
- Surgical: hernia repair is advisable for most patients with a groin hernia in order to reduce the risks of future complications. The most common approach for repair is still an open operation through the groin, although laparoscopic repair for recurrent, bilateral and unilateral inguinal hernias is increasingly common. In both cases a permanent synthetic mesh is implanted. Laparoscopic repair requires a general anaesthetic, while open repair can be performed under local anaesthetic.

Specifically, in the case of this 25-year-old, he should have his hernia repaired urgently on the next available theatre list.

CASE 1.2 – 'I can't push my lump back in anymore'

A1: What is the likely differential diagnosis?

- Inguinal hernia
- Femoral hernia
- Enlarged lymph node (infection, metastatic tumour)
- Femoral artery aneurysm
- Saphena varix

A2: What features of the given history support the diagnosis?

A previously reducible groin mass which is no longer so is a very clear history of a groin hernia. The patient's older age and chronic cough also support this.

A3: What additional features in the history would you seek to support a particular diagnosis?

Ask about urinary symptoms – benign prostatic hyperplasia (BPH) is common in this age group and increases the risk of post-operative acute urinary retention.

A4: What clinical examination would you perform and why?

Examine both groins and external genitalia. Perform a digital rectal examination (DRE) to exclude BPH.

A5: What investigations would be most useful and why?

Ultrasound may be useful to differentiate between clinically unclear entities.

A6: What treatment options are appropriate?

- Supportive: no role
- Medical: no role
- Surgical: early elective repair is indicated.

CASE 1.3 – 'My hernia is sore and I've started to vomit'

A1: What is the likely differential diagnosis?

- Inguinal hernia, with ischaemia and bowel obstruction
- Femoral hernia, with ischaemia and bowel obstruction
- Psoas abscess
- Infected lymph node

A2: What features of the given history support the diagnosis?

The recent change in the groin lump which has become more painful and the redness of the overlying skin indicate ischaemia of the hernia contents. Vomiting and constipation would suggest bowel obstruction. A femoral hernia is more likely to cause ischaemia as a result of the tight neck of the femoral canal.

A3: What additional features in the history would you seek to support a particular diagnosis?

It is necessary to exclude infections that would drain to the inguinal lymph nodes. Local inflammation could explain the erythema of the skin and tenderness of the lump. Systemic sepsis can secondarily cause paralytic ileus that would cause vomiting.

A4: What clinical examination would you perform and why?

Examine the groin carefully. Femoral hernias are seen more commonly in women than men, but an inguinal hernia is still more common in women than a femoral hernia. Femoral hernias are felt below and lateral to the pubic tubercle. Approximately 40 per cent of femoral hernias present with strangulation.

A5: What investigations would be most useful and why?

A plain abdominal x-ray will confirm the clinical suspicion of bowel obstruction. An arterial blood gas (ABG) test may show a metabolic acidosis and raised lactate, suggesting ischaemia. Other investigations will be directed at readying the patient for emergency surgery.

A6: What treatment options are appropriate?

- Supportive: no role
- Medical: the patient should be aggressively fluid resuscitated with the expectation of going to theatre urgently. Passing a nasogastric tube reduces the risk of vomiting and aspiration of gastric contents in addition to improving patient comfort.
- Surgical: emergency surgery is needed. This usually consists of a lower midline laparotomy, although other options are available. Any non-viable bowel will need to be resected, usually with an anastomosis of the two ends. The hernia itself can be repaired at the same time, either with a second groin incision, or from within the abdomen.

👥 OSCE Counselling cases

OSCE COUNSELLING CASE 1.1 – 'Should I have my hernia repaired?'

- Risks relate to the complications of the underlying condition as well as to the risks of any treatment.
- Risks of surgery may be due to the anaesthetic or the operation.
- Risks of an operation may be specific to that operation or general to all surgery.

General risks:

- Bleeding – minimized by careful surgical technique, stopping anticoagulation before surgery
- Wound infection
- Pain

Specific risks:

- Hernia recurrence
- Scrotal haematoma
- Injury to the vascular supply to the testicle (ischaemic orchitis and testicular atrophy)
- Chronic pain

Patients can only make informed choices about whether to proceed with surgical treatment if they are made aware of the risks of any treatment as well as the risks of the underlying condition if left untreated. There is strong consensus that groin hernias should usually be repaired.

OSCE COUNSELLING CASE 1.2 – 'Why did my surgeon suggest I see a urologist first?'

Q1: BPH is a relatively common condition in elderly men. Similar symptoms of bladder outflow obstruction can also be caused by prostate cancer. Most patients cope well with their symptoms, which are usually of gradual onset. Occasionally inguinal hernia repair may trigger acute urinary retention as a result of the combination of anaesthetic drugs, the perioperative fluid load given and pain in the groin. The treatment of acute urinary retention usually involves a urethral catheter, and may result in a prolonged hospital admission.

Q2: A urologist will take a detailed history, perform complete physical examination including DRE, and arrange further appropriate investigations. These may include a blood test for Prostate Specific Antigen (PSA), trans-rectal ultrasound of the prostate (TRUS) including prostate biopsy if necessary, and cystoscopy to assess the bladder and prostatic urethra. Medications may be all that are required to manage his symptoms. Trans-urethral resection of the prostate (TURP) may be appropriate. This assessment and treatment is best performed prior to uncomplicated elective hernia repair.

REVISION PANEL

- Hernias should usually be surgically repaired when present, in order to treat symptoms of discomfort, and to reduce the risk of serious complications.
- Ultrasound is sometimes required to diagnose atypical hernias (or hernias in unusual sites), and to exclude conditions that may mimic hernia, such as lymphadenopathy.
- Hernia repair may be open or laparoscopic. Each method has specific advantages and risks, which should be discussed with the patient. Neither has a fundamental advantage over the long term.
- Patients who present with bowel obstruction should be checked for hernia as a possible cause.
- Chronic pain is an under-recognized complication of hernia repair, and may occur in up to 10 per cent of patients.

GALLSTONES

Questions

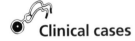 **Clinical cases**

For each of the clinical case scenarios given

Q1: What is the likely differential diagnosis?
Q2: What features of the given history support the diagnosis?
Q3: What additional features in the history would you seek to support a particular diagnosis?
Q4: What clinical examination would you perform and why?
Q5: What investigations would be most useful and why?
Q6: What treatment options are appropriate?

CASE 1.4 – 'My GP tells me my pain is caused by gallstones'

Right upper quadrant pain after fatty meals prompts a 26-year-old woman to see her GP. The pain is felt under the ribs and in her back. It builds up over an hour and lasts up to 4 hours. It is quite severe. She feels nauseated, but never vomits. The GP refers her for a surgical opinion, but suggests to her that the pain will probably turn out to be due to gallstones.

CASE 1.5 – 'It's the worst pain ever! It's not going away, and I've got a fever'

A 31-year-old woman has had typical biliary pain for many months, but has been reluctant to consider an operation. She now has an episode of constant pain that lasts 18 hours which she says is the worst ever. She looks flushed and has a temperature of 37.9°C. Nausea, and now vomiting are a feature.

CASE 1.6 – 'My eyes have gone yellow and my skin is itching'

A 61-year-old man has had niggling epigastric pain for some months. Over the last week his wife has commented that his eyes are yellow tinged. He has noticed that he is getting itchy skin.

👥 OSCE Counselling cases

OSCE COUNSELLING CASE 1.3 – 'But I don't have pain – do I need an operation?'

During an antenatal scan a 26-year-old woman is noted to have small mobile gallstones. When questioned she denies pain typical of biliary colic. She is referred by her obstetrician for a surgical opinion as to whether she should have a cholecystectomy.

Q1: Should she be offered an operation?

OSCE COUNSELLING CASE 1.4 – 'What is this ERCP thing that you think I should have?'

Six weeks after delivery the same young woman develops epigastric pain and jaundice. Ultrasonography confirms the presence of gallstones and shows a dilated common bile duct (CBD) of 11 mm. Endoscopic retrograde cholangiopancreatography (ERCP) is recommended.

Key concepts

In order to work through the core clinical cases in this chapter you will need to understand the following key concepts.

HOW DO GALLSTONES FORM?

Bile consists of water, sodium bicarbonate, bile salts, bile pigments, lecithin and cholesterol secreted by hepatocytes. Normally these constituents are in solution. Alterations in the relative amounts of these constituents can render bile 'lithogenic' (stone forming). Biliary infection, stasis and changes in gallbladder function can also cause precipitation around a nucleus of cellular debris or bacteria. Gallstones are formed.

WHAT CLINICAL PROBLEMS CAN THEY CAUSE?

Consider the problems by where the gallstones are located:

- Gallbladder: asymptomatic, biliary pain (colic), inflammation (cholecystitis), perforation, malignancy (75 per cent of gallbladder carcinoma is associated with stones)
- Bile ducts: asymptomatic, obstructive jaundice, ascending cholangitis, gallstone pancreatitis
- Unusual: fistula to duodenum, stomach or colon, gallstone ileus

WHAT OPTIONS ARE THERE FOR IMAGING THE BILIARY TREE?

Ultrasonography is usually the imaging investigation of choice for suspected gallstones. Ten per cent of gallstones are radio-opaque and visible on plain abdominal x-ray. ERCP gives excellent visualization of the lumen of the bile ducts, and also allows therapeutic interventions such as sphincterotomy, stone extraction and stent placement. Magnetic resonance cholangiopancreatography (MRCP) equals the imaging quality of ERCP but without the risks.

Answers

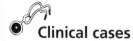

Clinical cases

CASE 1.4 – 'My GP tells me my pain is caused by gallstones'

A1: What is the likely differential diagnosis?
- Biliary colic
- Peptic ulcer disease

A2: What features of the given history support the diagnosis?
Pain associated with gallstones often occurs after fatty meals as the hormone cholecystokinin is released, causing the gallbladder to contract. As the stimulus is hormonal, the pain is usually of gradual onset but prolonged duration. Nausea is common. Referred pain is often felt in the back or shoulder.

A3: What additional features in the history would you seek to support a particular diagnosis?
A family history of gallstones may be present, but this may reflect learnt eating behaviours rather than a genetic tendency to form gallstones. Symptoms of gastro-oesophageal reflux and upper gastrointestinal bleeding should be sought.

A4: What clinical examination would you perform and why?
Abdominal examination should be performed, although often no signs are found. Check the eyes for jaundice. Note any abdominal scars that might make laparoscopic surgery more difficult.

A5: What investigations would be most useful and why?
- Ultrasonography to confirm the presence of gallstones and assess the bile ducts
- Blood tests to look for evidence of ductal calculi (raised bilirubin, alkaline phosphatase, amylase)

A6: What treatment options are appropriate?
- Supportive: adopting a low-fat diet may reduce the frequency and severity of attacks of biliary colic.
- Medical: medical options to dissolve gallstones have been tried unsuccessfully in the past.
- Surgical: most patients with symptomatic gallstones should have the gallbladder removed (cholecystectomy). Laparoscopic cholecystectomy can be performed successfully in 95 per cent of patients, with 5 per cent requiring open surgery (either planned open surgery, or due to an intra-operative decision to convert from a laparoscopic technique).

CASE 1.5 – 'It's the worst pain ever! It's not going away, and I've got a fever'

A1: What is the likely differential diagnosis?
- Acute cholecystitis
- Ascending cholangitis (obstructed CBD with infection ascending into the liver)
- Right lower lobe pneumonia
- Less likely: acute appendicitis, pyelonephritis, perforated peptic ulcer

A2: What features of the given history support the diagnosis?

Her past history of typical biliary pain, now superseded by constant prolonged pain and systemic upset suggest infection and inflammation of the gallbladder.

A3: What additional features in the history would you seek to support a particular diagnosis?

Exclude symptoms of any other infections – cough, urinary frequency. Ask about dark urine, pale stools and itching which suggest jaundice is present and makes ascending cholangitis a possibility.

A4: What clinical examination would you perform and why?

Abdominal examination may reveal tenderness and even peritonism in the right upper quadrant. Murphy's sign – the cessation of inspiration as the inflamed gallbladder descends onto the examining fingers in the right upper quadrant – is tested. Charcot's triad (jaundice, fever with rigors and right upper quadrant pain) indicate ascending cholangitis.

A5: What investigations would be most useful and why?

- Blood tests: elevated white cell count (WCC) is likely to be present. Electrolytes should be normal unless there is dehydration or prolonged vomiting present. Liver function tests (LFTs) may be mildly out of range, but high bilirubin or amylase suggests diagnoses other than acute cholecystitis.
- Ultrasonography: will confirm gallstones, and may identify features of acute cholecystitis – thickened gallbladder wall, pericholecystic fluid, the sonographic Murphy's sign. An abscess or gallbladder perforation should also be evident. In a severely ill patient, computed tomography (CT) may be more appropriate.

A6: What treatment options are appropriate?

- Supportive: fluid resuscitation and analgesia, including non-steroidal anti-inflammatory drugs (NSAIDs), are available.
- Medical: antibiotics have traditionally been used to resolve acute cholecystitis. Often a prolonged course (10 to 14 days) is required.
- Surgical: early laparoscopic cholecystectomy has been shown to be as safe as initial medical management with elective laparoscopic cholecystectomy 6 weeks later. The advantage of surgery during the initial admission is reduced hospital admissions and elimination of the risk of further complications while waiting for surgery.
- Other: in very sick patients, or those with significant comorbidity, percutaneous image-guided drainage of an empyema (pus-filled gallbladder) in addition to antibiotics is an option.

CASE 1.6 – 'My eyes have gone yellow, and my skin is itching'

A1: What is the likely differential diagnosis?

- Obstructive jaundice due to gallstones
- Obstructive jaundice due to malignancy (e.g. pancreatic carcinoma, enlarged metastatic lymph nodes, liver metastases)
- Jaundice from other causes

A2: What features of the given history support the diagnosis?

Pain from stones within the ductal system is often intermittent and difficult to characterize. Obstructive jaundice classically results in yellowing of the sclera and skin, dark urine and pale stools and intense itching. Weight loss associated with jaundice is a worrying sign of malignancy, often indicating advanced disease.

A3: What additional features in the history would you seek to support a particular diagnosis?

- Exclude other causes of jaundice: pre-hepatic and hepatic versus post-hepatic (obstructive)
- Any new medications?
- Blood transfusions?
- Sickle cell disease?

A4: What clinical examination would you perform and why?

Look for signs of liver failure, starting at the hands and working centrally. Check the supraclavicular fossa on the left for enlarged lymph nodes. Carefully examine the abdomen, particularly for masses.

A5: What investigations would be most useful and why?

- Blood tests: check the LFTs and check clotting (which is a good indicator of hepatic synthetic function).
- Imaging: start with ultrasonography, the simplest accurate way of detecting gallstones. Also CT or magnetic resonance imaging (MRI) are excellent at defining the site and characteristics of a mass. ERCP and MRCP can both image the bile ducts, but ERCP allows acquisition of brushings for cytology and therapeutic interventions as well. Endoscopic ultrasound is also useful to assess the pancreas and regional lymph nodes, and to take FNA samples for cytology.

A6: What treatment options are appropriate?

- Supportive: good hydration is important because patients with jaundice are more prone to renal impairment.
- Medical: antibiotics are often started as prophylaxis against ascending infection. Vitamin K can help to restore clotting function.
- Surgical: cholecystectomy, intra-operative imaging of the bile ducts using an image intensifier (cholangiography) and exploration of the CBD using a flexible camera (choledochoscopy) can allow removal of CBD stones at the same time as removing the gallbladder.
- Other: ERCP with stone extraction is often carried out before cholecystectomy is performed as definitive treatment. Small numbers of patients undergoing ERCP develop pancreatitis, perforation, bleeding or die as a result of the procedure.

ᴬᴬ OSCE Counselling cases

OSCE COUNSELLING CASE 1.3 – 'But I don't have pain – do I need an operation?'

Gallstones are common, affecting 20 per cent of women and 10 per cent of men in the United Kingdom. Only about 30 per cent of people with gallstones ever have symptoms or complications related to their gallstones. In most patients with gallstones, symptoms become gradually, rather than rapidly worse.

Only a small number of patients without symptoms should be advised to have their gallbladder removed – patients with a calcified gallbladder (risk of malignancy) on plain abdominal x-ray, diabetics (higher rates of complications if they develop cholecystitis) and those with sickle cell disease.

OSCE COUNSELLING CASE 1.4 – 'What is this ERCP thing that you think I should have?'

ERCP is a diagnostic and therapeutic procedure performed using a specialized side-viewing endoscope. The endoscope has channels through which instruments can be inserted and guided into the biliary tree. Radio-opaque dye can be injected in order to delineate the anatomy of the bile ducts and identify stones or strictures causing obstruction. Electrocautery can enlarge the sphincter of Oddi (sphincterotomy) and special baskets and crushing forceps can clear the duct of stones. Tumours can be biopsied, or brushings of the duct lining can be taken for cytology.

This procedure is highly specialized, and even in expert hands has a small failure rate. Complications are rare, but include bleeding or perforation (from sphincterotomy), pancreatitis in up to 3 per cent (probably due to high-pressure dye injection) and death in 0.5 per cent.

REVISION PANEL

- Gallstones are relatively common, and present in patients younger than traditionally reported.
- Gallstones may be asymptomatic or may cause pain (biliary colic), inflammation (cholecystitis), blockage (obstructive jaundice, ascending cholangitis, pancreatitis) or other complications.
- Diagnosis is primarily by ultrasound. Specific imaging of the biliary anatomy with ERCP or MRCP is indicated after pancreatitis, or if biochemical or clinical jaundice is present.
- Cholecystectomy should be performed for symptomatic gallstones. Acute cholecystectomy for cholecystitis and after pancreatitis has been shown to be safe in experienced surgical hands.
- Antibiotic treatment of cholecystitis, or drainage with a radiologically inserted cholecystostomy (drainage tube) may be considered when surgery is not possible.

APPENDICITIS

Questions

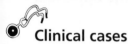

Clinical cases

For each of the clinical case scenarios given

> **Q1:** What is the likely differential diagnosis?
> **Q2:** What features of the given history support the diagnosis?
> **Q3:** What additional features in the history would you seek to support a particular diagnosis?
> **Q4:** What clinical examination would you perform and why?
> **Q5:** What investigations would be most useful and why?
> **Q6:** What treatment options are appropriate?

CASE 1.7 – 'I've got a really bad pain in my right side'

A 17-year-old man comes to the accident and emergency (A&E) department with a 12-hour history of nausea, lack of appetite and vague pain that is becoming more severe and localized to the right lower abdomen.

CASE 1.8 – 'I've developed another episode of pain on the right side'

Moderate right-sided lower abdominal pain has brought a 24-year-old woman to the surgical assessment unit. She has had this on two previous occasions, with no diagnosis made. The pain is constant, and is associated with nausea.

CASE 1.9 – 'The pain is getting worse and I've started to vomit'

A 45-year-old businessman has delayed coming to hospital and is now doubled over with severe pain, vomiting and rigors. When seen he is tachycardic and has a palpable abdominal mass in the right iliac fossa.

👥 OSCE Counselling cases

OSCE COUNSELLING CASE 1.5 – 'I'm going to overwinter in the Antarctic. Should I have my appendix removed beforehand?'

A 32-year-old male meteorologist is planning to spend 6 months at a research station in the Antarctic; this sometimes becomes inaccessible to medical evacuation flights for up to a month at a time. He has heard that sometimes prophylactic appendicectomy is performed in this situation.

Q1: What would you advise?

OSCE COUNSELLING CASE 1.6 – 'Why has my wife developed complications after her appendicectomy?'

After having her appendix removed last week, a 44-year-old woman has started to feel progressively more unwell, with lower abdominal pain, fevers and diarrhoea. Her GP sends her back into hospital, where a pelvic abscess is diagnosed on abdominal CT.

Q1: What will you tell this woman about why this has happened?

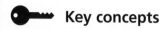 **Key concepts**

In order to work through the core clinical cases in this section you will need to understand the following key concepts.

WHAT IS APPENDICITIS?

Inflammation of the appendix is usually caused by obstruction of the lumen by a faecolith (a small hard ball of faecal material), with subsequent stasis, distal distension, bacterial overgrowth, venous engorgement and subsequent impairment of the blood supply, necrosis of the wall and finally perforation if not treated promptly.

The peak incidence of appendicitis is in the second and third decades, with a second peak in the seventh decade.

WHAT HAPPENS IF THE APPENDIX PERFORATES?

The risk of perforation within 24 hours of the onset of symptoms is <30 per cent, and perforation occurs more commonly in children.

The omentum tends to wall off serosal inflammation of the appendix. Perforation may be contained by the omentum and other surrounding structures to form a localized abscess. If this does not happen, generalized peritonitis is likely.

Answers

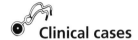

Clinical cases

CASE 1.7 – 'I've got a really bad pain in my right side'

A1: What is the likely differential diagnosis?

- Acute appendicitis
- Gastroenteritis
- Mesenteric adenitis
- Crohn's disease of the terminal ileum
- Less likely: ureteric colic, acute cholecystitis, pyelonephritis

A2: What features of the given history support the diagnosis?

Appendicitis is typically preceded by a vague abdominal pain, because visceral inflammation is often poorly localized to the midline; organs derived from the midgut usually have pain referred to the periumbilical region. As the serosa becomes inflamed, and involves the peritoneum, the pain tends to localize to where the appendix is located. Nausea and anorexia go hand in hand with gastrointestinal (GI) inflammation.

A3: What additional features in the history would you seek to support a particular diagnosis?

Has the patient had this type of pain previously? Recurrent pains are atypical of appendicitis ('grumbling' appendix, while much beloved of GPs, probably does not exist). Ask about other GI symptoms, particularly diarrhoea; in appendicitis, these usually follow the initial pain, rather than preceding it. Also check for family history of inflammatory bowel disease, and recent viral infections.

A4: What clinical examination would you perform and why?

Abdominal examination should seek to differentiate between tenderness (mild to moderate pain on palpation) and guarding (increased muscular tone) which is a sign of peritonism. Cough and percussion tenderness are hallmarks of peritonism, and when present with the appropriate history are often diagnostic of acute appendicitis. Rebound tenderness is non-specific and cruel, and should never be performed.

In most patients with suspected acute appendicitis DRE adds little information.

Repeated clinical assessment is very useful in borderline cases. A 12-hour period of assessment with repeated examination is almost always safe, and better than operating in the middle of the night.

A5: What investigations would be most useful and why?

- Blood tests: In acute appendicitis, WCC and inflammatory markers (C-reactive protein (CRP)) are usually moderately raised. Other blood tests are normal.
- The presence of UTI can be excluded by midstream urine (MSU).
- Plain abdominal x-ray adds little. Computed tomography of the right iliac fossa is highly sensitive and specific for appendicitis, but is not usually required.

A6: What treatment options are appropriate?

- Supportive: no role
- Medical: broad-spectrum antibiotics can alter the course of early appendicitis, but once serosal inflammation or ischaemia/necrosis of the wall has occurred, the appendix will progress to perforation if not removed. Antibiotics can be given as prophylaxis against wound infection at the time of anaesthetic induction, or as a course of post-operative treatment if the appendix has perforated.
- Surgical: appendicectomy is indicated. This can be performed as an open operation with an incision in the right iliac fossa, or laparoscopically (see next section).

CASE 1.8 – 'I've developed another episode of pain on the right side'

A1: What is the likely differential diagnosis?

- Non-specific abdominal pain
- Acute appendicitis
- Right-sided gynaecological pathology (ovarian cyst rupture or torsion, pelvic inflammatory disease, ectopic pregnancy, endometriosis, midcycle ovulatory pain)
- Less likely: Crohn's disease, gastroenteritis, cholecystitis or biliary colic, ureteric colic

A2: What features of the given history support the diagnosis?

The previous episodes of the same pain suggest a recurring problem, although it is possible to have similar episodes before frank acute appendicitis.

A3: What additional features in the history would you seek to support a particular diagnosis?

Could she be pregnant? A careful gynaecological and sexual history is mandatory in this situation. Urinary symptoms should also be elicited.

A4: What clinical examination would you perform and why?

In addition to abdominal examination, vaginal and pelvic examination should be performed. Masses, tenderness, vaginal discharge and cervical excitation should all be sought.

A5: What investigations would be most useful and why?

- Perform a pregnancy test before anything else.
- Blood tests: Obtain WCC, haemoglobin (Hb), urea and electrolytes (U&Es) and CRP.
- Collect MSU to exclude UTI.
- Imaging: traditionally ultrasonography (transvaginal being better than transabdominal) has been used to assess right iliac fossa pain in young women. However, this frequently fails to achieve a diagnosis.
- Diagnostic laparoscopy: use if pain fails to resolve after a period of overnight observation, and other tests have not achieved a diagnosis. It has the benefit of allowing direct visualization of the appendix and pelvic organs, and the ability to proceed to therapeutic intervention if necessary.

A6: What treatment options are appropriate?

- Supportive: fluids, analgesia and a period of observation are useful when the diagnosis is equivocal. Those with mild pain which resolves may then eat and drink and be discharged without follow-up.
- Medical: there is no role, although antibiotics should be started once a diagnosis of appendicitis has been made if there is going to be a delay in getting to theatre.

- Surgical: surgery is indicated for definite signs of acute appendicitis. It is generally accepted that removing a normal appendix ('negative appendicectomy') is less dangerous than equivocating and allowing the appendix to perforate, an abscess to form, or generalized peritonitis to develop.

CASE 1.9 – 'The pain is getting worse and I've started to vomit'

A1: What is the likely differential diagnosis?

- Appendix abscess
- Appendix mass
- Perforated ileal Crohn's disease
- Perforated caecal cancer

A2: What features of the given history support the diagnosis?

This story is typical of 'missed' appendicitis; patients usually present to hospital within 24 to 48 hours of symptoms starting. If the appendix perforates, systemic signs of sepsis (tachycardia, tachypneoa, pyrexia) are often more severe.

A3: What additional features in the history would you seek to support a particular diagnosis?

GI symptoms that have been present for a long period may point to underlying pathology such as inflammatory bowel disease. Neoplasms may be asymptomatic in the caecum as a result of the liquid stool and large calibre of the caecal lumen, but may result in iron-deficiency anaemia and consequent lethargy.

A4: What clinical examination would you perform and why?

Abdominal examination should be performed to confirm the presence of a tender right iliac fossa mass. It may also be felt on DRE.

A5: What investigations would be most useful and why?

- Blood tests: raised WCC, raised CRP. Iron-deficiency anaemia may suggest a caecal malignancy. In systemic sepsis, LFTs can be deranged (raised alanine aminotransaminase (ALT) and aspartate aminotransaminase (AST) and reduced albumin).
- Imaging: plain abdominal x-ray may show signs of an ileus or frank bowel obstruction. Plain erect chest x-ray may show free gas under the diaphragm if bowel perforation has occurred. Ultrasound or CT of the abdomen must be performed urgently to differentiate an appendix mass from an appendix abscess, or to diagnose an underlying caecal malignancy or features of Crohn's disease, as these clinical entities will be managed differently.

A6: What treatment options are appropriate?

- Supportive: fluid resuscitation and analgesia are needed.
- Medical: if an appendix mass (without an abscess) is diagnosed, broad-spectrum antibiotics targeted against GI organisms should be given. If the patient settles with this treatment, only 20 per cent develop recurrent appendicitis. Performing an 'interval' appendicectomy is no longer recommended. Any underlying bowel pathology should be excluded by either colonoscopy or CT colonography in patients over the age of 40.
- Radiological: if a localized appendix abscess is present, ultrasound or CT-guided percutaneous drainage should be performed, and may avoid the need for an operation.

- Surgical: surgery will be required if the inflammation is localized (appendicectomy via the usual right iliac fossa incision or midline laparotomy), or if generalized peritonitis is present (midline laparotomy to allow appendicectomy and washout of the abdominal cavity). Perforated Crohn's disease or caecal cancer may require laparotomy and resection of the affected bowel segment. Rejoining the bowel may be unwise in the presence of infection, so a temporary stoma may be necessary.

ᴀ̊ᴀ̊ OSCE Counselling cases

OSCE COUNSELLING CASE 1.5 – 'I'm going to overwinter in the Antarctic. Should I have my appendix removed beforehand?'

Appendicitis affects between 7 and 12 per cent of individuals in their lifetime, most often in the second and third decades. The risk for any individual in a given 6-month period is relatively small, and impossible to predict. The risk of complications associated with removing a normal appendix must be weighed against the risks of developing appendicitis when access to medical care might be difficult.

Laparoscopic appendicectomy has reduced the risk of complications and morbidity associated with the operation, and most surgeons would at least consider such a request in appropriate circumstances.

OSCE COUNSELLING CASE 1.6 – 'Why has my wife developed complications after her appendicectomy?'

All medical interventions have the potential to cause harm as well as good. Informed consent should include information about common adverse events, as well as rare but significant complications. Patients should always have the opportunity to ask as much about their care as they feel appropriate. This is sometimes harder to do in an emergency situation.

Pelvic abscess is an uncommon but recognized complication of appendicitis. Appropriate medical care, including antibiotics and drainage should minimize the risk of long-term sequelae.

REVISION PANEL

- Appendicitis is a common cause of the acute abdomen in younger patients.
- The diagnosis of appendicitis is primarily a clinical assessment. Pregnancy should *always* be excluded in females of childbearing age.
- Sometimes CT scanning or other imaging may be required to obtain the diagnosis in equivocal cases. Examples include the elderly, or when a mass is present.
- Surgical treatment is preferred for acute appendicitis. Diagnostic laparoscopy followed by laparoscopic (or open) appendicectomy is now commonly performed, particularly in women.
- A macroscopically normal appendix may sometimes be left in situ with a laparoscopic approach, especially if other pathology is identified. A normal appendix should *never* be left in place after an open appendicectomy incision has been made.

COLON AND RECTAL CANCER

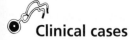

Clinical cases

For each of the clinical case scenarios given

> **Q1:** What is the likely differential diagnosis?
> **Q2:** What features of the given history support the diagnosis?
> **Q3:** What additional features in the history would you seek to support a particular diagnosis?
> **Q4:** What clinical examination would you perform and why?
> **Q5:** What investigations would be most useful and why?
> **Q6:** What treatment options are appropriate?

CASE 1.10 – 'I've developed rectal bleeding'

A 45-year-old woman has intermittently noticed some dark liquid blood and occasional blood clots in her bowel motions over the last 3 months. She is otherwise well and her bowel habit has not altered.

CASE 1.11 – 'My bowel habit has changed'

The 48-year-old husband of the same woman mentions that he is troubled by not passing a motion as frequently as usual, and when he does, sometimes it is looser. He once noticed some bright red blood on the toilet paper. He is worried because his older brother developed bowel cancer when he was in his late forties.

CASE 1.12 – 'It feels like I can't finish my bowel motion'

A 74-year-old man has been complaining of intermittent colicky abdominal pains with frequent dark blood in the stools. Over the last 2 months he has noticed that he feels 'funny' deep inside his pelvis when he passes a motion, and never feels like he has completely emptied (tenesmus). His trousers have become looser and he has had to punch another hole in his belt.

👥 OSCE Counselling cases

OSCE COUNSELLING CASE 1.7 – 'What do I need to know about colonoscopy?'

The 45-year-old woman mentioned above had a colonoscopy organized, and was anxious about the procedure. She understood the need for the test, but heard that it was very painful.

Q1: What are the risks of colonoscopy?

OSCE COUNSELLING CASE 1.8 – 'Why are they talking about radiotherapy before my bowel cancer operation?'

A 66-year-old man with rectal bleeding and tenesmus is found to have a large fixed mass on rectal examination. Biopsies confirm rectal cancer and MRI shows probable metastatic nodes in the mesorectum. A referral for pre-operative radiotherapy is made.

Q1: What does radiotherapy add?
Q2: Are there any side effects that the patient needs to know about?

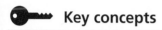 **Key concepts**

In order to work through the core clinical cases in this section you will need to understand the following key concepts.

WHAT IS THE DIFFERENCE BETWEEN COLONIC AND RECTAL CANCER?

Although the underlying disease process is the same – neoplastic epithelial cells lining the large bowel – they present with a different spectrum of symptoms as a result of their different anatomical sites. In the right colon, huge growth can occur with little in the way of symptoms, and iron-deficiency anaemia is common. In the left colon, dark but noticeable bleeding may be the most common symptom. Low rectal cancers, near the anus, in the confined space of the pelvis, may cause brighter bleeding or defecation symptoms (e.g. tenesmus, a feeling of incomplete evacuation).

Surgery and other treatments may differ markedly according to the site of the tumour: radiotherapy is often used in the pelvis for rectal cancer, whereas chemotherapy may be used for advanced colon cancer.

WHAT CAUSES COLON CANCER?

There is a well-defined pathway from normal colonic epithelium, to dysplastic changes in the cells, to early neoplasia (such as benign adenomatous polyps) and subsequently to true malignancy – the adenoma-carcinoma sequence. This pathway suggests that finding and treating benign polyps early may reduce the risk of later cancer. This is the basis of the bowel screening programme.

WHAT ARE THE PRINCIPLES OF TREATMENT OF COLORECTAL CANCER?

The aim of treatment should obviously be curative in most cases, and the mainstay of treatment is surgical resection. Where this is not possible because distant metastasis has already occurred, local control of disease remains important. Obstruction and bleeding are the most important local complications of colorectal cancer, and stenting, resection of the affected segment and interventional radiological techniques to embolize bleeding vessels is usually appropriate. Chemotherapy and radiotherapy are important treatment modalities in specific situations; multidisciplinary assessment should be the rule rather than the exception.

Answers

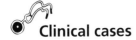

Clinical cases

CASE 1.10 – 'I've developed rectal bleeding'

A1: What is the likely differential diagnosis?
- Haemorrhoids
- Proctitis/colitis
- Bleeding from a polyp or cancer

A2: What features of the given history support the diagnosis?

With a history of rectal bleeding that is not typically haemorrhoidal (e.g. bright red, painless, only occurring with defecation) in a patient over the age of 40, other sources of the bleeding need to be considered and excluded. The lack of other symptoms makes serious pathology less likely, but remember that early colorectal cancer may have few symptoms.

A3: What additional features in the history would you seek to support a particular diagnosis?

Ask about other alterations in bowel habit. Is there a family history of bowel cancer? If sinister causes for the bleeding are ultimately excluded, a careful dietary history may reveal too little fibre in the diet – a common theme in minor anorectal conditions.

A4: What clinical examination would you perform and why?

Abdominal examination including a DRE is critical. Masses should be sought, and identified when present. Feel for hepatomegaly. Check the conjunctiva for pallor. Proctoscopy and rigid sigmoidoscopy should be performed in the outpatient clinic if the equipment is available.

A5: What investigations would be most useful and why?

If the index of suspicion for malignancy is low, rigid sigmoidoscopy to examine the rectum, followed by flexible sigmoidoscopy (to examine the left colon), colonoscopy (to examine the whole colon) or CT colonography should be performed. The benefit of endoscopic procedures is the ability to take biopsies and remove polyps, while CT avoids the potential complications associated with these therapeutic interventions. Barium enema is rarely used in current practice.

In the case of this lady, colonoscopy was performed and showed four small polyps scattered throughout the colon, and one 2-cm pedunculated lesion in the distal left colon.

A6: What treatment options are appropriate?

With the therapeutic ability of colonoscopy, the polyp was removed with a diathermy snare cauterizing through the stalk. The polyp was retrieved and sent for histology, showing it to be a dysplastic polyp with no evidence of malignancy.

If the polyp had been shown to be malignant, further treatment options would include endoscopic mucosal resection or surgical resection of the involved segment of colon. Being benign, one should consider the need for further colonic surveillance in the future – developing polyps makes future polyps more likely. Current guidelines suggest repeat colonoscopy at 1 year if high risk, 3 years if intermediate risk and 5 years if low risk for developing colorectal cancer, determined by the size and number of adenomatous polyps found.

CASE 1.11 – 'My bowel habit has changed'

A1: What is the likely differential diagnosis?

- Diverticular disease
- Colitis
- Left-sided colon cancer

A2: What features of the given history support the diagnosis?

Alteration of the bowel habit over the age of 40 is always significant, but benign causes such as diverticular disease are more common than malignancy. Bleeding has not been a major feature, and neither has tenesmus. The family history of colorectal cancer is worthy of note, although the cancer risk associated with a single first-degree relative under the age of 50 is less than 1 in 12 (three to six times baseline population risk).

A3: What additional features in the history would you seek to support a particular diagnosis?

Ask about other non-colonic cancers in the family history which may raise the possibility of hereditary non-polyposis colorectal cancer (HNPCC), such as endometrial, ovarian, gastric and pancreatic. Ask about weight change.

A4: What clinical examination would you perform and why?

Abdominal examination, DRE, proctoscopy and rigid sigmoidoscopy

A5: What investigations would be most useful and why?

Colonoscopy is the most useful investigation in this situation, although abdominal CT and CT colonography are becoming much more commonly used. Biopsy can be performed at colonoscopy if suspicious masses or polyps are encountered.

In this man's case CT colonography was performed and identified significant sigmoid diverticulosis. The report commented that small polyps within the sigmoid colon could not be completely excluded by the examination. As a result, he underwent flexible sigmoidoscopy subsequently, and no further abnormality was found.

A6: What treatment options are appropriate?

- Supportive: as there has been no complication of the diverticular disease, dietary management (with a high-fibre diet) may reduce the risk of progression of this acquired condition. Many patients will, however, ultimately progress and require specific treatments.
- Medical: antibiotics may be required for the infective complications of diverticular disease, either diverticulitis or the development of a peri-diverticular abscess. The latter of these may also require image-guided percutaneous drainage. Free perforation with generalized peritonitis usually requires an emergency operation.
- Surgical: resection of the affected bowel segment (usually the sigmoid colon) may be required in some patients, usually those with repeated hospitalization or complications. Severe diverticulitis with perforation may require emergency surgery, either with a Hartmann procedure (sigmoid colectomy with end colostomy; this may be joined up 6 to 12 months later) or resection and primary anastomosis.

CASE 1.12 – 'It feels like I can't finish my bowel motion'

A1: What is the likely differential diagnosis?

- Rectal cancer
- Left-sided colon cancer
- Severe diverticular disease

A2: What features of the given history support the diagnosis?

This history sounds ominous: the 'funny' feeling is called tenesmus and is characteristic of advanced rectal cancer. Weight loss with the other features described is an important symptom.

A3: What additional features in the history would you seek to support a particular diagnosis?

Again, a family history should be obtained. A thorough history and systems enquiry will be required as a major operation may be required.

A4: What clinical examination would you perform and why?

Abdominal and rectal examination, with proctoscopy and rigid sigmoidoscopy should be performed. This reveals a large hard rectal mass, and the liver is palpable and craggy. General examination is required to detect any other significant findings.

A5: What investigations would be most useful and why?

A number of investigations are necessary. Biopsy of the mass can be performed in clinic. Then CT of the thorax, abdomen and pelvis will be required to assess for distant metastatic disease, and MRI of the pelvis will be necessary to assess suitability for surgical resection. Endoanal ultrasound may also play a part in assessing the possibility of resection. Colonoscopy will be required to assess the rest of the colon for other polyps or tumours (synchronous lesions).

A6: What treatment options are appropriate?

- Supportive: nutrition is important and should be optimized. When there is widespread disease, or when the patient declines surgical treatment, palliative care measures such as pain relief are of critical importance.
- Medical: little role
- Surgical: surgery is undertaken with either curative or palliative intent. Resection can either be performed through the abdomen (anterior resection of the rectum), or via a combined approach taking out the tumour and the anal canal in the perineum (abdominoperineal resection of the rectum). In the first case, a temporary protective ileostomy may be formed, in the latter there will be a permanent end-colostomy. This may be done even in the presence of liver metastases in order to minimize symptoms in the future. In some patients, resection of the liver metastases is also performed.
- Other: radiotherapy to the tumour in the pelvis may be performed as an extra treatment combined with surgery, and may be done to shrink the tumour before surgery (neo-adjuvant radiotherapy) or to reduce the incidence of local recurrence after surgery (adjuvant radiotherapy). If the tumour cannot be excised, or the patient declines surgery, primary treatment with radiotherapy may provide palliative benefit. Chemotherapy has a limited role in rectal cancer.

⚥ OSCE Counselling cases

OSCE COUNSELLING CASE 1.7 – 'What do I need to know about colonoscopy?'

Colonoscopy is usually a safe procedure, but a number of issues need to be discussed. These relate to the risks of the procedure itself, and the risks of the sedation that usually accompanies colonoscopy.

The oral bowel cleansing agents that are used to clear out the colon prior to examination can be unpleasant; they cause diarrhoea and can result in dehydration and electrolyte disturbance. Clear written and verbal instructions should be given prior to their use.

Perforation is extremely rare with diagnostic colonoscopy, but rises (still uncommon) with interventional procedures such as polypectomy. Perforation is usually treated with antibiotics and active observation. Surgery is rarely required. Death from colonoscopy is almost unheard of. Significant bleeding is also very rare.

Failure of the procedure to visualize the entire colon should be discussed. Completion rates, with identification of the caecum and often intubation of the terminal ileum, exceed 95 per cent in experienced hands. Despite excellent technique, lesions are sometimes missed.

OSCE COUNSELLING CASE 1.8 – 'Why are they talking about radiotherapy before my bowel cancer operation?'

Q1: Pre-operative (neo-adjuvant) radiotherapy is used either where tumour shrinkage ('down-staging') is required to convert a borderline resectable tumour into one that can confidently be removed, or to minimize the risks of local recurrence in operable but advanced disease (i.e. invasion through the rectal wall, or nodal involvement on imaging). A number of trials have now shown that radiotherapy reduces local recurrence and improves survival when used appropriately.

Q2: Radiotherapy risks can be considered as general and site specific. Common general side effects include tiredness and a local skin reaction similar to sunburn.

Site-specific radiotherapy complications in the pelvis may include vaginal dryness in women, and impotence in men. The latter may respond to medical treatments such as sildenafil (Viagra). Most radiotherapy avoids the gonads and should not impair fertility. However, sperm banking is an option some may want to consider. Bladder or bowel inflammation can occur with radiotherapy, and to some degree, the latter is inevitable. This can cause bleeding, diarrhoea and incontinence. A diverting colostomy is sometimes required.

Late complications can also occur, and should be carefully discussed with the radiation oncologist.

REVISION PANEL

- Rectal bleeding should always be taken seriously, and investigated appropriately.
- Abdominal examination, DRE, proctoscopy and sigmoidoscopy should be performed in all patients with rectal bleeding or any suspicion of colorectal cancer.
- Colonic examination with either radiological imaging (double contrast barium enema or CT colonography) or colonoscopy is usually required. Colonoscopy has the advantage of allowing biopsy if pathology is identified.
- Colorectal cancer should be managed by experts. Rectal cancer in particular requires urgent specialist investigation and treatment, sometimes including pre-operative radiotherapy or chemotherapy before an operation.
- Diverticular disease is common in Western society, and may be treated non-operatively in many circumstances. Occasionally, emergency operation is required for complications such as perforation.

SURGICAL EMERGENCIES

Questions

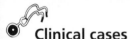

Clinical cases

For each of the clinical case scenarios given

> **Q1:** What is the likely differential diagnosis?
> **Q2:** What features of the given history support the diagnosis?
> **Q3:** What additional features in the history would you seek to support a particular diagnosis?
> **Q4:** What clinical examination would you perform and why?
> **Q5:** What investigations would be most useful and why?
> **Q6:** What treatment options are appropriate?

CASE 1.13 – **An acute abdomen**

A 70-year-old man is brought into A&E complaining of abdominal pain. Over the last few months he has noted a change in his bowel habit and loss of weight. On examination he is pale, tachycardic and hypotensive and his abdomen is rigid on palpation.

CASE 1.14 – **Bowel obstruction**

A 60-year-old woman presents with a 2-day history of abdominal distension, pain, profuse bilious vomiting and constipation.

Answers

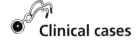
Clinical cases

CASE 1.13 – **An acute abdomen**

A1: What is the likely differential diagnosis?

This man has an acute abdomen. The most likely underlying diagnosis is perforated viscus (peptic ulcer, acute appendicitis, caecal cancer, sigmoid diverticular disease, perforated gallbladder). Other common causes include acute pancreatitis, ischaemic bowel, ruptured abdominal aortic aneurysm (AAA) and non-surgical causes (myocardial infarction, diabetic ketoacidosis and lower lobe pneumonia).

A2: What features of the given history support the diagnosis?

The age of the patient, recent change in bowel habit and weight loss suggest a left-sided colonic neoplasm. The sudden onset of severe pain could indicate a perforation, probably at the site of the tumour, or at the caecum if the tumour has caused large bowel obstruction and the ileocaecal valve is competent (this causes a closed-loop obstruction). Right iliac fossa pain and tenderness may be a warning sign of impending perforation in such cases and requires urgent action. Severe diverticular disease can cause colonic perforation, but does not usually cause weight loss. Free gas on an erect chest x-ray and an acute abdomen are also seen in perforated duodenal or gastric ulcer disease. This is normally accompanied by a history of peptic ulcer disease or ingestion of NSAIDs, and the patient tends to be less septic than in faecal peritonitis.

A3: What additional features in the history would you seek to support a particular diagnosis?

Other factors that would point towards a colonic cancer include history of passing blood mixed with stool, a family history of bowel cancer and related cancers and previous colon cancer or inflammatory bowel disease.

A4: What clinical examination would you perform and why?

A full examination should be undertaken. Abdominal examination will assess which quadrant of the abdomen is most tender, and may demonstrate the palpable pulsatile mass in the upper abdomen consistent with a ruptured AAA. A rectal tumour may be revealed by DRE and should always be performed. A rigid, silent abdomen would suggest generalized peritonitis.

A5: What investigations would be most useful and why?

Blood: full blood count (FBC) may reveal anaemia secondary to bleeding from the tumour. An indication of the degree of metabolic acidosis would be given by ABG. Clotting parameters and LFTs may be abnormal in the severely septic patient. Amylase and blood glucose levels should be checked in all patients with an acute abdomen.

Imaging: an erect chest x-ray should be performed and may show free gas under the diaphragm. It should be remembered that its absence does not rule out perforation. If the patient is stable and the diagnosis is equivocal, urgent abdominal CT should be performed.

A6: What treatment options are appropriate?

- Supportive: high-flow oxygen should be given via a face mask. The patient should be aggressively fluid resuscitated with several litres of crystalloid, and a urinary catheter sited to monitor urine output and guide fluid management. A wide-bore nasogastric tube should be inserted if the patient is vomiting. Opiate analgesia should be given regularly. Thromboembolic deterrent stockings (TEDs) should be applied, and low-molecular-weight heparin given after discussion with the anaesthetist, depending upon whether the plan is to insert an epidural catheter for post-operative pain management.
- Medical: broad-spectrum antibiotics should be given. This patient requires surgery to treat the problem, but every effort should be made to optimize his condition prior to surgery. This is best achieved in a critical care environment.
- Surgery: a Hartmann's procedure (sigmoid colectomy, closure of the rectal stump, and end colostomy) would be the safest option for a sigmoid perforation. An alternative to this would be resection of the affected colon, on-table washout, and primary anastomosis. This avoids the need for a stoma and secondary reversal procedure, but has the risk of anastomotic breakdown and leak.

Faecal peritonitis carries a high mortality rate, and good communication with the patient and family should ensure that they are aware of this before surgery.

CASE 1.14 – **Bowel obstruction**

A1: What is the likely differential diagnosis?

The most likely diagnosis is bowel obstruction (probably small bowel). The most common causes would be hernias, adhesions, malignancy and volvulus.

A2: What features of the given history support the diagnosis?

The classic symptoms of small bowel obstruction (SBO) are those given in the history: pain, distension, bilious vomiting and constipation. If the vomiting were feculent and intermittent, large bowel obstruction would be suspected. (This requires an incompetent ileocaecal valve to allow backflow.)

A3: What additional features in the history would you seek to support a particular diagnosis?

The aim of the history is to determine the level of obstruction (e.g. proximal SBO causes profuse frequent bilious vomiting and minimal distension, and patients may still be opening their bowels) and the cause. A history of previous abdominal surgery, particularly for malignancy, could be very important.

A4: What clinical examination would you perform and why?

Abdominal examination may reveal the presence of an irreducible hernia. Severe localized tenderness is a sign of impending perforation in a closed-loop obstruction. Bowel sounds may be hyperactive early in SBO, becoming tinkling and eventually absent as time progresses.

A5: What investigations would be most useful and why?

- Blood tests: ABG may show a metabolic acidosis due to dehydration, or if the bowel's blood supply is compromised. Due to a co-existing metabolic alkalosis due to vomiting, ABG can be difficult to interpret. Due to acute kidney injury, U&Es may be deranged.
- Imaging: a plain abdominal x-ray will show dilated small bowel loops, occasionally with an obvious cut-off point. A contrast follow-through, or CT with oral contrast will be useful in determining the level of obstruction, and if adhesions are the cause, may give prognostic information about whether the obstruction is likely to resolve without the need for surgery.

A6: What treatment options are appropriate?

- Supportive: fluid resuscitation is essential because of the large volume of fluid lost into the bowel lumen (third space loss). A wide-bore nasogastric tube will decompress the bowel, relieve vomiting, and give an indication as to whether the obstruction has resolved.
- Medical: no role
- Surgical: in a patient with no history of previous abdominal surgery, where there is physiological or biochemical evidence of bowel ischaemia, or in whom an irreducible hernia has been found, surgery should be performed after optimization. In those with suspected adhesional obstruction and no clinical evidence of bowel ischaemia, a period of fluid resuscitation and nasogastric drainage ('drip and suck') can be undertaken to allow spontaneous resolution.

REVISION PANEL

- Patients who present with an acute abdomen need urgent assessment with simultaneous resuscitation and treatment.
- The most useful radiological investigation is CT if the patient is stable enough to be safely transported to a radiology department.
- Peritonitis, particularly from hollow viscus perforation, is a disease with a high morbidity and mortality rate.
- Most patients with an acute abdomen will require an expeditious laparotomy to conclusively identify and manage the underlying pathology. Principles of treatment include relief of obstruction, resection of pathology, washout and dilution of soiling, repair or anastomosis of bowel when safe to do so and consideration of stoma formation when not.

VASCULAR: ABDOMINAL AORTIC ANEURYSM

Questions

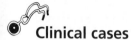

Clinical cases

For each of the clinical case scenarios given

> **Q1:** What is the likely differential diagnosis?
> **Q2:** What features of the given history support the diagnosis?
> **Q3:** What additional features in the history would you seek to support a particular diagnosis?
> **Q4:** What clinical examination would you perform and why?
> **Q5:** What investigations would be most useful and why?
> **Q6:** What treatment options are appropriate?

CASE 1.15 – 'I thought I had gallstones. What is an aneurysm?'

A 65-year-old male publican was sent by his GP for ultrasonography for suspected gallstones. The report shows no gallstones, but comment is made about a 4.5-cm abdominal aortic aneurysm.

CASE 1.16 – 'My doctor tells me I need an operation on my aneurysm'

The same patient has regular scans. Three years later the aneurysm has grown to 6 cm. He is referred to a vascular surgeon; she recommends an operation to repair the aneurysm.

CASE 1.17 – Severe back pain and collapse with a known aneurysm

A patient in the same practice is also known to have an aneurysm, measuring 6 cm in diameter. He was reluctant to have an operation. He has had back pain for 2 days, which became severe this morning. Visiting the practice for pain relief, he suddenly becomes clammy, yells in pain and collapses. An ambulance is called.

👥 OSCE Counselling cases

OSCE COUNSELLING CASE 1.9 – 'What about this "stenting" I've heard about?'

A 57-year-old woman with a 5.5-cm abdominal aortic aneurysm has had treatment recommended to her. She does an Internet search and finds that there is an alternative to open surgery, where the aneurysm is stented from inside the vessel, with almost immediate recovery. Can she have this treatment?

OSCE COUNSELLING CASE 1.10 – 'It's not that serious. I couldn't die from this operation could I?'

As part of the counselling and consent process, a patient becomes very concerned that he might die from the operation. Surely this can't be common?

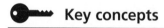 **Key concepts**

In order to work through the core clinical cases in this section you will need to understand the following key concepts.

DEFINITION OF AN ANEURYSM

An *aneurysm* is a permanent, localized and abnormal dilatation (>1.5 times normal) of a blood vessel. A true aneurysm involves all vessel wall layers (artery – intima, media, adventitia), whereas a false aneurysm (pseudo-aneurysm) is a haematoma that forms as a result of a leaking hole in an artery (usually iatrogenic – arterial puncture, site of anatomises) and is contained by the surrounding tissues. This differs from an arterial dissection, in which there is separation of the arterial wall layers.

RISK FACTORS FOR AN ABDOMINAL AORTIC ANEURYSM

- *Age* – most commonly seen in people aged >60-years-old
- *Smoking* – strong risk factor for the development of an aortic aneurysm
- *High blood pressure* – damages the blood vessel wall
- *Male gender* – men more commonly develop aortic aneurysms
- *Atherosclerosis* – can damage and weaken the arterial wall
- *Ethnicity* – more common in white populations
- *Family history* – people with a family history of aortic aneurysms tend to have a higher incidence, develop them at a younger age and are at a higher risk of rupture

The presence of popliteal or femoral aneurysms is a warning sign; they often co-exist.

WHAT IS THE NATURAL HISTORY?

The expansion rate of aneurysms is variable in individual patients, but most will enlarge at 0.5 cm per annum for aneurysms below 4.9 cm and 0.7 cm per annum for those between 5 and 5.9 cm. Aneurysms below 5.5 cm in diameter are unlikely to rupture and patients are generally observed with ultrasound. In aneurysms beyond 5.5 cm, the risk of rupturing is usually greater than the risk of having it repaired.

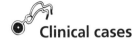

Answers

Clinical cases

CASE 1.15 – 'I thought I had gallstones. What is an aneurysm?'

A1: What is the likely differential diagnosis?

Although the diagnosis is clear in this case, the aetiology has a differential diagnosis. Most aneurysms are degenerative, but rarely infection (mycotic aneurysms), trauma, pancreatitis, and connective tissue disorders (Marfans, Ehlers-Danlos) can be predisposing factors.

A2: What features of the given history support the diagnosis?

Male sex, age over 65, hypertension and smoking are the most important risk factors.

A3: What additional features in the history would you seek to support a particular diagnosis?

Other manifestations of cardiovascular disease include coronary artery disease and peripheral vascular disease (PVD), both of which have classic symptoms. There is a high rate of aneurysms in siblings (especially brothers) and this should be asked about.

A4: What clinical examination would you perform and why?

A full cardiovascular, respiratory and peripheral vascular examination should be performed including BP measurement. Clinical examination should include careful and gentle palpation of the abdomen – an aneurysm is characterized by 'expansile pulsation' (where the examining fingers of both hands move laterally apart as well as anteriorly in time with the pulse). Aneurysms may also occur in the same patient in the iliac, femoral and popliteal arteries, so these should also be checked.

A5: What investigations would be most useful and why?

For active surveillance (which would be appropriate in this case), ultrasonography is cheap, accurate and reproducible and does not involve exposure to radiation. Its main disadvantages are that it is observer dependent and visualization of the suprarenal aorta and iliac arteries may be difficult. The study may also prove impossible in the grossly obese or when large amounts of bowel gas are present. Other investigations should be aimed at predisposing factors. An ECG, cholesterol, blood glucose and renal function should be assessed.

A6: What treatment options are appropriate?

For a small aneurysm (<5.5 cm), observation is appropriate with 6 to 12 monthly ultrasound scans. The frequency of measurement is increased closer to 5-cm diameter and if there is a rapid increase in size between scans. This 'watchful waiting' is appropriate as the risk of rupture in small aneurysms (~1 per cent per year at 4-cm diameter versus 10 per cent per year at 6 cm) is considerably lower than the risk of surgery. Risk factor management is vital in such patients including controlling hypertension, hyperlipidaemia, diabetes and weight. Patients should be started on aspirin, statin and appropriate antihypertensive medication.

CASE 1.16 – 'My doctor tells me I need an operation on my aneurysm'

A1: What is the likely differential diagnosis?

As for Case 1.15.

A2: What features of the given history support the diagnosis?

As for Case 1.15.

A3: What additional features in the history would you seek to support a particular diagnosis?

As for Case 1.15.

A4: What clinical examination would you perform and why?

As for Case 1.15.

A5: What investigations would be most useful and why?

A CT scan should be performed to assess the maximal size, the configuration of the aneurysm and importantly whether the origins of the renal arteries are involved (suprarenal aneurysm) or normal (infrarenal aneurysm). The former is less common but poses a much more complex problem. Information from the scan can also be used to determine the suitability of the aneurysm to being repaired endovascularly (a stent deployed from within the artery through incisions in the groin), see A6. More extensive assessment of fitness for surgery should be undertaken to ensure the patient is as fit as possible (e.g. cardiac stress test, respiratory function tests, cardiac echocardiography and up-to-date blood tests).

A6: What treatment options are appropriate?

There is a 40 per cent chance of rupture over the next 5 years and the average survival without treatment is about 18 months. Options should be chosen with this in mind.

- Conservative treatment with risk factor modification may be advised, either at patient request or if the anaesthetic and operative risks are thought to outweigh the benefits.
- Open operation: the aneurysmal segment of the aorta is replaced with a synthetic (Dacron) graft by laparotomy. Death from this operation occurs in 5 to 8 per cent of patients and has an overall complication rate of 15 to 20 per cent.
- Endovascular stenting: this is a more recently developed technique; expanding stents are introduced via the femoral arteries and deployed from aorta to iliac arteries within the aneurysm sac, excluding the aneurysm and preventing further growth and risk of rupture. This method is only suitable in approximately 50 per cent of cases due to anatomical constraints.

  Endo-leaks (a persistent blood flow outside the lumen of the endoluminal graft but within an aneurysm sac) are common and if considered significant require re-intervention. The long-term results are not known as the technology of the graft materials is constantly progressing (although results are encouraging) and patients are subjected to a lifetime of surveillance which although improving can involve significant doses of radiation from frequent CT scans.

CASE 1.17 – Severe back pain and collapse with a known aneurysm

A1: What is the likely differential diagnosis?

Rupture of the aneurysm is most likely and must be assumed.

Other intra-abdominal catastrophes that may mimic a ruptured aneurysm include a perforated gastric/duodenal ulcer, pancreatitis, renal colic, appendicitis, cholelithiasis and right-sided heart failure with pulsatile hepatomegaly.

A2: What features of the given history support the diagnosis?

The prodromal pain of a contained leak is not uncommon. In the face of a known aneurysm, acute severe abdominal or back pain demands immediate attention.

A3: What additional features in the history would you seek to support a particular diagnosis?

It is unlikely that further history taking in this emergency situation would be helpful. A history from a family member may be useful to ensure that inappropriate surgery is not attempted (e.g. if the patient has an advanced incurable malignancy).

A4: What clinical examination would you perform and why?

Clinical examination in this setting may reveal a pulsatile mass, but the absence of such a finding should not dissuade emergency investigation and treatment. It is not uncommon for the abdomen to be rigid. Examination of the patient's cardiovascular stability is important to determine the urgency of surgery over further resuscitation and investigation.

A5: What investigations would be most useful and why?

Rapid ultrasound scanning (FAST-scan) by trained A&E doctors can often give the diagnosis of a ruptured abdominal aortic aneurysm. Emergency CT may be considered if the patient is stable to confirm diagnosis or assess suitability for endovascular repair, but this should be only on the request of the operating vascular surgeon. All patients should have blood taken for cross-matching according to unit protocol (usually 6 to 10 units of blood, plus fresh frozen plasma (FFP)).

A6: What treatment options are appropriate?

Initial management should *not* include aggressive fluid resuscitation because this may lead to greater blood loss by displacing any clot at the site of rupture. A systolic pressure of 90 to 100 mm Hg is optimum and ensures cerebral perfusion pressure. The only effective treatment for a ruptured abdominal aortic aneurysm is emergency repair. Rupture is highly lethal: as a rule of thumb, about half of patients die at the scene, half of the remainder die en route to hospital or in A&E, and half of those who make it to theatre will subsequently die.

Laparotomy and open repair is still the mainstay of surgical treatment, but in stable patients who have a CT scan confirming favourable anatomy and with the appropriate expertise, endovascular repair of ruptured aneurysms is possible.

OSCE Counselling cases

OSCE COUNSELLING CASE 1.9 – 'What about this "stenting" I've heard about?'

Aortic stenting involves a vascular surgeon and/or radiologist inserting an expandable covered tube into the inside of the weakened and dilated aortic wall through small incisions in the groins either under general or regional anaesthesia. Placement is assisted using radiological guidance. Although it can have a quicker recovery and is less invasive than open surgical treatment, stenting is only suitable in approximately half of patients who require surgery due to anatomical constraints. Although the technology of the materials is constantly improving, the long-term outcomes are not known. In addition, some new complications of leakage around the graft (endo-leaks) are recognized and occasionally require re-intervention with further surgery. There is a risk of rupture during the procedure so patients must be warned that a conversion to open surgery may be required. After surgery, patients will be kept in a surveillance programme to observe the aneurysm size and graft placement, which may require repeated exposure to radiation.

OSCE COUNSELLING CASE 1.10 – 'It's not that serious. I couldn't die from this operation, could I?'

Depending on a number of factors, around 5 to 8 per cent of patients die from elective abdominal aortic aneurysm repair, and important complications occur in around 15 to 20 per cent of patients. Both morbidity and mortality figures can be modified – excellent surgeons in excellent centres may achieve very good results, but selecting lower-risk patients will also appear to give the same outcome.

Any operative and anaesthetic risk should be weighed against the risk of the disease itself. A 6-cm aneurysm has about a 40 per cent risk of rupture over 5 years, and the median survival of a group of patients with such an aneurysm is around 18 months.

REVISION PANEL

- Aneurysmal dilatation of major arteries is an important condition to identify and treat. When found, other manifestations of arterial disease should be sought.
- Once an aneurysm is discovered, appropriate further investigations should be determined by a specialist vascular surgical service.
- Treatment options and thresholds are continuing to evolve. In particular, aneurysm stenting is a technique with increasing use.
- Aortic aneurysm rupture must always be suspected in the appropriate setting (i.e. acute severe abdominal pain, with or without hypotension). This is a true surgical emergency, and the best option is sometimes taking the patient directly to an operating theatre without investigation. If ruptured aneurysm is considered a possibility, *discuss with a surgeon immediately.*

PERIPHERAL VASCULAR DISEASE (PVD)

Questions

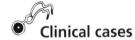

Clinical cases

For each of the clinical case scenarios given

> **Q1:** What is the likely differential diagnosis?
> **Q2:** What features of the given history support the diagnosis?
> **Q3:** What additional features in the history would you seek to support a particular diagnosis?
> **Q4:** What clinical examination would you perform and why?
> **Q5:** What investigations would be most useful and why?
> **Q6:** What treatment options are appropriate?

CASE 1.18 – **A 78-year-old man presents complaining of calf pain on walking**

CASE 1.19 – **The same man presents to A&E with an acutely painful leg**

Key concepts

In order to work through the core clinical cases in this section you will need to understand the following key concepts.

NATURAL HISTORY OF PVD

- The prevalence of asymptomatic PVD is 7 to 15 per cent.
- Intermittent claudication affects 5 per cent of patients over the age of 50.
- Approximately 75 per cent of patients with claudication will remain stable or improve.
- Approximately 5 per cent of patients with claudication will progress to critical ischaemia every year.
- Approximately 1 to 2 per cent will require a major amputation.
- Absolute coronary heart disease risk in claudicants is 30 per cent over 10 years. Patients with PVD have a 25 per cent greater likelihood of mortality than patients without PVD.

CRITICAL LEG ISCHAEMIA

This is defined as rest pain for more than 2 weeks, or ulceration/gangrene, and an ankle pressure of <50 mm Hg or a toe pressure of <30 mm Hg.

Pain is often worse at night when the feet are in the supine position and the cardiac output and BP are decreased during sleep. The patient often hangs his or her leg out of bed or sleeps in a chair.

RISK FACTORS FOR PVD

- *Age* – PVD increases with age in both men and women.
- *Smoking* – the most important modifiable risk factor for PVD is smoking.
- *Diabetes* – diabetics have an up to 2.5 times greater risk of PVD than non-diabetics.
- *Hypertension* – this is present in up to 50 per cent of patients with PVD.
- *Cholesterol* – patients with PVD benefit from statin therapy, with increased pain-free walking distance and quality of life.

VASCULAR IMAGING

Non-invasive imaging using duplex ultrasound scanning (combined ultrasonography and Doppler colour flow images), MR angiography (MRA) and CT angiography (CTA) has now superseded digital subtraction angiography due to improved quality of the imaging and safety.

Digital subtraction angiography (DSA) is performed by a catheter inserted into the femoral vessels (usually the contralateral vessel to allow retrograde insertion of the catheter into the aortic bifurcation). It is now usually only carried out as a combined procedure to allow angioplasty or stent insertion to improve blood flow. It has a small but significant complication rate when associated with non-invasive imaging, is expensive, time consuming and often requires an overnight stay tying up hospital beds.

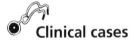

Answers

Clinical cases

CASE 1.18 – **A 78-year-old man presents complaining of calf pain on walking**

A1: What is the likely differential diagnosis?

- Peripheral vascular disease
- Spinal stenosis or sciatica

A2: What features of the given history support the diagnosis?

The most likely cause will be PVD caused by atherosclerosis to the vessels of the lower limbs. The site of stenosis or occlusion will affect the presenting symptoms. The proximal disease (e.g. common iliac) may produce buttock claudication on exercise as well as lower limb pain. The most common site to be affected is the obturator foramen (two-thirds of the way down the thigh). This produces classic intermittent claudication (IC). The important aspects to obtain are the distance walked before having to stop (remember that most patients and doctors are poor at judging this and that the distance will be longer on the flat rather than uphill), the time required for the pain to resolve and walking to recommence and an assessment of the nature of the problem (static or progressive).

Spinal stenosis causes a similar presentation, making differentiation between the two sometimes tricky. Lower limb pain from spinal stenosis tends to occur after varying distances and does not resolve within minutes of rest (unlike in IC). The subsequent distances may become shorter and the time for resolution of the pain increases. The patient may also complain of a 'bad' back with neurological symptoms.

A3: What additional features in the history would you seek to support a particular diagnosis?

The diagnosis may be supported by the fact that the individual has risk factors that predispose him to atherosclerosis and he may have other cardiovascular problems.

A4: What clinical examination would you perform and why?

A full cardiovascular and peripheral vascular examination should be performed. The lower limbs may show signs of muscle wasting, thinning of skin and loss of hair. Peripheral pulses may be felt in the groin but are absent distally. Gangrene and tissue loss (ulceration) would indicate critical ischaemia, a stage beyond intermittent claudication.

A5: What investigations would be most useful and why?

In an individual not showing signs of critical ischaemia or disabling claudication the investigations undertaken would be aimed at preventing disease progression and not treating the stenosis or occlusion. Bloods including full-blood count (for anaemia), U&Es, fasting cholesterol and random blood glucose. Ankle brachial pressure indices (ABPIs) may be recorded to allow quantitative comparison of future follow-up. But the majority of patients with stable claudication do not require any further investigation and are followed up clinically.

A6: What treatment options are appropriate?

Cardiac function should be optimized to decrease any 'pump failure' as a cause. Strategies to slow disease progression should be undertaken (cessation of smoking, statins, antiplatelet medication, good diabetic control and treatment of hypertension).

Regular exercise improves neovascularization and cardiorespiratory function and helps in weight loss. A structured exercise program is proven to improve outcomes for claudicants.

CASE 1.19 – The same man presents to A&E with an acutely painful leg

A1: What is the likely differential diagnosis?

The patient appears to have developed acute limb ischaemia. This is commonly the result of either thrombosis of the diseased vessels or an embolus occluding the vessel. In a known sufferer of PVD, the most likely cause is thrombosis.

A2: What features of the given history support the diagnosis?

Remember the 6 P's of acute limb ischaemia – pale, pulseless, painful, paralysed, paraesthetic and 'punishingly cold'.

A3: What additional features in the history would you seek to support a particular diagnosis?

An acute thrombosis due to a ruptured atheromatous plaque is the likely diagnosis in this patient who has a chronic history of intermittent claudication. Acute thrombosis of a popliteal aneurysm may present with an acutely ischaemic leg. Patients may have a history of a popliteal aneurysm or have other aneurysmal disease present in the popliteal or femoral arteries and the abdominal aorta. Embolus should be considered in patients who have no previous PVD history, or who have normal pulses on the opposite leg. A source of emboli should be considered, such as patients with new onset atrial fibrillation or a recent myocardial infarction.

A4: What clinical examination would you perform and why?

An examination will need to assess the viability of the limb and the urgency for intervention. Sensory and motor function should be assessed and recorded. If the diagnosis is in doubt, ABPIs can be performed. The patient's general state should be assessed because acute limb ischaemia is often a pre-morbid episode and surgical intervention may cause unnecessary suffering.

If considering bypass surgery, the peripheral veins should be noted (varicosities) as these are typically used for bypass grafts.

A5: What investigations would be most useful and why?

Imaging of the arterial anatomy with either CT angiogram or MR angiogram if time permits would be indicated. An on-table angiogram may be performed if radiologists are present. Duplex USS may also be used if more detailed imaging is not and can also be useful in determining the venous anatomy for a suitable conduit (but should not delay theatre).

In embolic cases, the source of emboli should be investigated using ECG, echocardiography or duplex for abdominal aortic aneurysm.

A6: What treatment options are appropriate?

Depending on the suitability, a bypass graft may be attempted to restore flow. If the limb is unsalvageable then an amputation may be required.

Patients who are very frail may not be suitable for any intervention and should be made comfortable.

VASCULAR: CAROTID

Questions

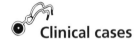 **Clinical cases**

For each of the clinical case scenarios given

> **Q1:** What is the likely differential diagnosis?
> **Q2:** What features of the given history support the diagnosis?
> **Q3:** What additional features in the history would you seek to support a particular diagnosis?
> **Q4:** What clinical examination would you perform and why?
> **Q5:** What investigations would be most useful and why?
> **Q6:** What treatment options are appropriate?

CASE 1.20 – **A 72-year-old man is referred to the vascular surgeons with a spontaneously resolving right-sided weakness and difficulty speaking**

Duplex ultrasound revealed a 90 per cent stenosis of his internal carotid artery.

CASE 1.21 – **A previously well 39-year-old man attends A&E with a left-sided headache and slight word-finding difficulty after a mild whiplash injury 2 hours earlier**

He says the right arm does not 'feel right'. His wife has noticed a slight drooping of the left eyelid.

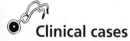

Answers

Clinical cases

CASE 1.20 – **A 72-year-old man is referred to the vascular surgeons with a spontaneously resolving right-sided weakness and difficulty speaking**

A1: What is the likely differential diagnosis?

- Likely diagnosis is of a transient ischaemic attack (TIA) involving the left middle cerebral artery (MCA)
- Migraine with aura
- Epilepsy
- Cerebral haemorrhage
- Brain tumour
- Hypoglycaemia

A2: What features of the given history support the diagnosis?

The transient nature of the weakness – TIA is defined as a neurological deficit due to cerebral ischaemia lasting less than 24 hours. Classical carotid territory symptoms include hemisensory or hemimotor symptoms, transient monocular blindness (Amaurosis Fugax) and higher cortical dysfunction (dysphasia, visual-spatial neglect).

A3: What additional features in the history would you seek to support a particular diagnosis?

Identify a history of peripheral vascular disease risk factors (BP, diabetes mellitus, cholesterol, smoking, family history of stroke/PVD).

A4: What clinical examination would you perform and why?

A full neurological, cardiac and peripheral vascular examination should be performed to identify signs of residual neurology or neurological deficit not consistent with a carotid territory TIA (i.e. vertebrobasilar symptoms – gait, stance, bilateral motor/sensory symptoms, diplopia, vertigo, nystagmus).

Examine for a cardiac source of emboli such as atrial fibrillation, mural thrombus or endocarditis. A carotid bruit may be present with a tight internal carotid artery stenosis.

A5: What investigations would be most useful and why?

A CT head should be performed to exclude an intracranial cause such as haemorrhage or tumour. Carotid duplex is the most commonly used modality for evaluating the degree of internal carotid artery stenosis. If an alternative to duplex is required to investigate the aortic arch vessels or intracerebral vessels, MR angiogram and CT angiogram have largely superseded catheter angiography.

A6: What treatment options are appropriate?

Initial treatment by the referring clinician should be to ensure the patient is on 'best medical therapy', a statin, antiplatelet, good diabetic control and if required anti-hypertensives.

The current 'gold standard' is a carotid endarterectomy to remove the embolizing internal carotid artery stenosis.

Carotid artery stenting has developed as an alternative to open surgery over the last 15 years. However, results have shown surgery to still be the safest form of intervention to prevent future risk of stroke.

CASE 1.21 – A previously well 39-year-old man attends A&E with a left-sided headache and slight word-finding difficulty after a mild whiplash injury 2 hours earlier

A1: What is the likely differential diagnosis?

- Most likely is dissection of the left carotid artery
- Left-sided intracerebral haemorrhage
- Migraine with aura
- Cerebrovascular disease causing a left-sided stroke in the MCA territory

A2: What features of the given history support the diagnosis?

Carotid artery dissection is a significant cause of stroke in patients younger than 40 years. Dissections are usually subadventitial (between the media and adventitia or within the media), creating a false lumen that can cause stenosis, occlusion or pseudoaneurysm of the vessel. Simultaneously, the dissection may cause the formation of thrombus from which fragments embolize. Strokes resulting from carotid dissection thus may have a haemodynamic or embolic origin.

As in this case, carotid artery dissections have non-specific presenting symptoms such as neurological deficits and headache. They often occur at a relatively young age and in previously healthy individuals, either spontaneously or after various degrees of trauma.

In this case a major clue to the cause of this patient's stroke is that he has a painful drooping left eyelid that suggests the possibility of Horner's syndrome. Horner's syndrome is caused by damage to the sympathetic supply to the eye. The sympathetic fibres travel with the carotid artery and carotid dissection may damage their blood supply. A Horner's syndrome consists of ipsilateral ptosis, miosis, enopthalmos and sometimes loss of sweating. It is important to consider a carotid dissection in any case of painful Horner's syndrome.

The patient is very young to have significant cerebrovascular disease. The other causes mentioned would not generally be expected to cause a Horner's syndrome, but remain possibilities.

A3: What additional features in the history would you seek to support a particular diagnosis?

If the patient does not have a previous or family history of migraine this reduces the possibility of a migrainous aetiology.

A4: What clinical examination would you perform and why?

Signs of an upper motor neuron pattern of sensory-motor deficit in the right arm and signs of a Horner's syndrome (see above) should be found. It is also important to search for evidence of a head injury and given the history of neck pain, to exclude evidence of a spinal fracture (cervical spine tenderness) and spinal cord damage (bilateral limb weakness and sensory loss).

A5: What investigations would be most useful and why?

- CT/MRI brain
- CT/MR angiography or invasive angiography
- Duplex ultrasonography of the carotid artery

Computed tomography of the brain will be adequate in most circumstances to demonstrate ischaemic damage in the MCA distribution, although MRI is more sensitive. Duple ultrasonography of the carotid arteries is fast, convenient, non-invasive and highly sensitive, and may identify a dissection. Invasive angiography is more accurate but carries greater risk than non-invasive alternatives including CTA and MRA. ECG and echocardiography may be performed to rule out a cardiac source of embolus.

A6: What treatment options are appropriate?

- Aspirin
- Anticoagulation

The majority are treated conservatively with heparinization and then warfarinization, with the aim being to reduce thrombosis or embolization. Surgery is usually reserved for those who have significant narrowing of the lumen of the artery or recurrent neurological events. Dissection carries a 20 per cent mortality and an even higher rate of persistent neurological disability.

VENOUS DISEASE

Questions

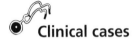 **Clinical cases**

For each of the clinical case scenarios given

Q1: What is the likely differential diagnosis?
Q2: What features of the given history support the diagnosis?
Q3: What additional features in the history would you seek to support a particular diagnosis?
Q4: What clinical examination would you perform and why?
Q5: What investigations would be most useful and why?
Q6: What treatment options are appropriate?

CASE 1.22 – A 65-year-old woman has noticed a breakdown in the skin over her left lower leg

The lower limb is swollen and discoloured.

Key concepts

In order to work through the core clinical cases in this section you will need to understand the following key concepts.

WHAT IS AN ULCER?

An ulcer is a lesion on the surface of the skin or mucous surface resulting in epi-/endothelial loss produced by the sloughing of inflammatory necrotic tissue.

WHAT ARE THE POSSIBLE AETIOLOGIES OF AN ULCER ON THE LOWER LEG?

- Venous disease
- Arterial disease
- Neuropathy (e.g. secondary to diabetes)
- Malignancy
- Underlying osteomyelitis
- Inflammatory (e.g. pyoderma gangrenosum)
- Vasculitis

Venous ulceration is a result of an increase in venous pressure of the lower limb. Over time this leads to changes seen in the 'gaiter' area of the leg. Chronic venous insufficiency is a term used to describe these changes, which are characterized by pigmentation, lipodermatosclerosis (thickening of the skin), swelling, varicose eczema and ulceration. The cause of this increased pressure is abnormalities to the flow caused by incompetent veins either due to previous deep vein thrombosis (DVT) or varicosities of the superficial long and short saphenous veins.

Answers

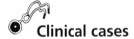 **Clinical cases**

CASE 1.22 – **A 65-year-old woman has noticed a breakdown in the skin over her left lower leg**

A1: What is the likely differential diagnosis?

See above.

A2: What features of the given history support the diagnosis?

Ulceration over the lower limbs is a common problem with venous ulceration accounting for about 1 per cent of the National Health Service (NHS) budget.

Approximately 80 per cent of patients presenting with ulcers will have evidence of venous disease. Up to 25 per cent will have Doppler-detected arterial disease and approximately 15 per cent will have co-existent diabetes and/or rheumatoid arthritis. It is therefore not uncommon to have ulcers of mixed aetiology.

With chronic skin changes (discolouration) and lower limb swelling and the fact that venous disease is the most common, this patient is likely to have venous ulceration.

A3: What additional features in the history would you seek to support a particular diagnosis?

Minor injury often precipitates the ulceration, the initial wound failing to heal and slowly deteriorating into an ulcer. A history of varicose veins with possible previous surgery and/or a family history of chronic venous insufficiency may be present. There may be a history of previous DVT or undiagnosed leg swelling in the past (occult DVT). Identify any history of diabetes, rheumatoid arthritis, vasculitis, renal impairment or steroid use.

A4: What clinical examination would you perform and why?

A full arterial, venous and neurological examination of the lower limb will assess the presence or absence of significant arterial and venous disease and or the presence of peripheral neuropathy.

Venous ulceration typically occurs around the gaiter area of the lower leg and may be circumferential. The ulcer is often shallow with granulation and slough in the base and a heavy exudate. Arterial ulcers may occur in the gaiter area, but also on the foot and between toes. They are usually smaller and deeper, with a 'punched out' appearance, and may have a necrotic base sometimes with tendon or muscle exposed.

A5: What investigations would be most useful and why?

A non-invasive assessment of the venous system of the lower limbs should be performed. This will assess the deep vein patency and competence as well as the saphenofemoral, saphenopopliteal and perforator competence. This assessment is nearly always conducted with duplex ultrasound either in a specialist vascular lab or by the surgeon in clinic. Tourniquets and Doppler are now reserved almost exclusively for medical exams.

ABPI assessment is essential in all patients with ulceration to either exclude or identify the presence of arterial disease. (They may require compression.) If there is any suggestion of arterial disease or if an ulcer is not responding to treatment, MR or CT angiography should be used.

If an atypical ulcer, consider a biopsy (vasculitic, Marjolin's ulcer).
Assess oedema.

A6: What treatment options are appropriate?

Initial treatment will involve compression of the lower limb with four-layer compression bandages. Leg elevation is recommended when sitting or lying. Surgery should be considered in those with a patent deep venous system who have incompetence of the saphenofemoral, saphenopopliteal and or perforators.

Patients are best managed by specialist nurse-led ulcer clinics in the community, unless there are concerns of infection or rapid deterioration which may require hospital intervention.

Nutritional and vitamin supplementation may be required as well as optimization of medical problems. Patient education is essential to reduce recurrence.

BREAST

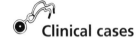
Clinical cases

For each of the clinical case scenarios given

Q1: What is the likely differential diagnosis?
Q2: What features of the given history support the diagnosis?
Q3: What additional features in the history would you seek to support a particular diagnosis?
Q4: What clinical examination would you perform and why?
Q5: What investigations would be most useful and why?
Q6: What treatment options are appropriate?

CASE 1.23 – 'I've found a breast lump'

You are asked to see a 24-year-old marketing manager who noticed a lump in her left breast 6 weeks ago. She has not had breast lumps previously, and has no family history of breast cancer. Examination reveals a 2-cm-diameter firm mass lateral to her left nipple.

CASE 1.24 – 'Something has shown up on my screening mammogram'

A 50-year-old woman is recalled for further assessment after her first-round screening mammograms show some 'calcifications'. Physical examination is unremarkable, with no lump palpable. A mammographic-guided stereotactic core biopsy is performed, and histology shows ductal carcinoma in situ (DCIS). Appropriate treatment needs to be arranged.

CASE 1.25 – 'I've found a lump under my armpit'

This 62-year-old woman sees her GP after noticing a hard lump under her right arm, and is referred urgently to a symptomatic breast clinic. The finding is confirmed, and also a hard 4-cm mass is felt in the right breast deep to the nipple. The clinical impression is one of breast cancer. Mammographic and ultrasound images support the diagnosis, and image-guided core biopsy of the breast mass and fine-needle aspiration of the axillary mass confirms malignant cells. Treatment options are discussed.

👫 OSCE Counselling cases

OSCE COUNSELLING CASE 1.11 – **'What can I do about this breast pain?'**

OSCE COUNSELLING CASE 1.12 – **'I'm confused about my surgical options for breast cancer. Which should I choose?'**

🔑 Key concepts

In order to work through the core clinical cases in this section you will need to understand the following key concepts.

HOW COMMON IS BREAST CANCER?

Breast cancer accounts for approximately 25 per cent of all female malignancies in the United Kingdom. Young women are much less likely to develop it, with the risk slowly increasing with age. The incidence is approximately 1 in 100 000 at age 40, rising to 400 in 100 000 at age 80. You may read that 1 in 8 to 12 women will get breast cancer. This is the cumulative, lifetime risk, which is age dependent.

'MY GRANDMOTHER HAD BREAST CANCER – WILL I GET IT TOO?'

There are a number of factors which will increase any given individual's risk of developing breast cancer. Hereditary breast cancers, caused by genetic abnormalities (e.g. the BRCA 1 or 2 genes) are responsible for only 10 per cent of all breast cancers. Other risk factors are much more common, but variable. Family history is important when it is a first-degree relative (mother or sister) and when the cancer was diagnosed pre-menopause, or has been diagnosed in multiple relatives. With a relatively common disease such as breast cancer, having more distant relatives with breast cancer is usually just chance.

HOW IS BREAST CANCER MANAGED?

Options for the diagnosis and treatment for breast cancer have expanded hugely over recent years. Management should occur within a multidisciplinary setting, involving radiologists, surgeons, pathologists, oncologists, specialist breast care nurses, and reconstructive surgeons in order to ensure the best outcomes for patients.

Answers

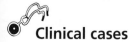

Clinical cases

CASE 1.23 – 'I've found a breast lump'

A1: What is the likely differential diagnosis?

- Fibroadenoma
- Fat necrosis
- Breast abscess
- Phyllodes tumour
- Breast cancer – less likely, but needs to be excluded

A2: What features of the given history support the diagnosis?

The young age of the patient makes the diagnosis of fibroadenoma the most likely, with other benign lesions also possible. Breast cancer in this age group is extremely rare, but needs to be considered; a strong family history would increase one's concern.

A3: What additional features in the history would you seek to support a particular diagnosis?

Ask about trauma to the breast, a history of which may support a diagnosis of fat necrosis. Also ask about breastfeeding, and medical conditions that would make infection more likely, including smoking.

A4: What clinical examination would you perform and why?

Clinical examination of both breasts, axillae and supraclavicular fossae should be performed with a chaperone present.

A5: What investigations would be most useful and why?

To complete the 'triple assessment', *imaging* and *biopsy* would normally be performed. Mammography is difficult to interpret in the dense breasts of women under the age of 40, and is only performed if a cancer is diagnosed. Ultrasound has greater diagnostic accuracy and is the imaging modality of choice in this age group. In the case of this 24-year-old woman, most breast surgeons would not biopsy this lesion if it felt typical of a fibroadenoma, and had the typical ultrasound appearances. Image-guided core biopsy could be performed if she was over 25, or there were any atypical features on examination or ultrasound.

A6: What treatment options are appropriate?

The natural history of fibroadenomas is that about a third spontaneously regress over time, one-third remain unchanged and one-third continue to grow. Women should understand this in order to make treatment choices.

- Non-operative: a significant proportion of women are adequately reassured by a benign diagnosis, and prefer to avoid an operation.
- Operative: removal of a fibroadenoma is usually possible with a small incision at the areolar margin, which normally results in a small, cosmetically acceptable scar.

CASE 1.24 – 'Something has shown up on my screening mammogram'

A1: What is the likely differential diagnosis?

Small flecks of calcium, seen on mammograms, are relatively common. Their likely diagnosis depends upon their shape, size and number. Large calcifications are usually not associated with cancer. Some configurations of calcium deposition are considered pathognomonic, such as cup-shaped dependent calcium in cysts. In contrast, groups of small calcifications ('clustered microcalcifications') may be associated with extra breast cell activity, usually benign, but sometimes in areas of early invasive cancer or DCIS.

A2: What features of the given history support the diagnosis?

Roughly 50 per cent of breast cancers in the United Kingdom are diagnosed before they have formed a lump through the mammographic screening programme. Screening is designed to identify DCIS or invasive breast cancer *early* to allow earlier, less radical treatments. Despite current controversies regarding the possible overtreatment of some women with subclinical disease which would have never caused symptoms, most large studies have shown screening is effective on a population basis.

A3: What additional features in the history would you seek to support a particular diagnosis?

Family history should again be determined for both breast and ovarian cancer. Although this will make no difference for this patient, it may have implications for her children.

A4: What clinical examination would you perform and why?

Examination of both breasts is required, in addition to complete physical examination.

A5: What investigations would be most useful and why?

The screening mammograms should be reviewed in the multidisciplinary meeting, and further views performed if required. Any previous screening films should be reviewed and audited to assess whether the lesion was visible earlier. An ultrasound scan of the axilla should be performed to assess for any abnormal looking lymph nodes.

As the lesion is not palpable, a mammographic stereotactic or ultrasound-guided core biopsy should be obtained.

Subsequent histological analysis of the stereotactic core biopsy shows DCIS.

A6: What treatment options are appropriate?

Treatment options for most women with DCIS are wide local excision and radiotherapy (breast-conserving therapy) if well localized and small, or if extensive or multifocal, mastectomy. To aid excision of an impalpable lesion, a wire is placed under mammographic or ultrasound guidance so that the tip lies adjacent to the area needing removal. Axillary staging with sentinel lymph node (SLN) biopsy is not performed for DCIS treated by breast-conserving therapy as the risk of axillary nodal spread is very small. If a mastectomy is being performed to treat DCIS, most surgeons would 'stage' the axilla with SLN biopsy. This is because there is a small risk of there being undiagnosed invasive breast cancer within a large area of DCIS, and also because SLN biopsy cannot be performed after mastectomy if an invasive breast cancer is found within the mastectomy specimen.

If a wide local excision is performed, the surgical margins need to be carefully assessed to ensure complete excision. Further excisions may be required to achieve this. In high-grade or extensive DCIS there is good evidence from large randomized trials that radiotherapy reduces the rate of local recurrence. Because 50 per cent of local recurrences after treatment for DCIS are invasive, initial optimal treatment is vital. Immediate reconstruction should be offered to any undergoing a mastectomy to treat DCIS.

CASE 1.25 – 'I've found a lump under my armpit'

A1: What is the likely differential diagnosis?

The diagnosis is secure – breast cancer with axillary lymph node metastasis. Attention should now be directed towards the presence of symptoms or signs of distant metastatic spread.

A2: What features of the given history support the diagnosis?

See above.

A3: What additional features in the history would you seek to support a particular diagnosis?

See above.

A4: What clinical examination would you perform and why?

Complete physical examination should search for metastases.

A5: What investigations would be most useful and why?

Investigations should be focussed on staging the disease and determining risk factors for anaesthesia and surgery. A CT scan of the thorax, abdomen and pelvis, and whole skeleton bone scan would be routine in this clinical setting.

A6: What treatment options are appropriate?

Unless the patient chooses a non-operative approach, surgery is required and is usually supplemented by chemotherapy, radiotherapy and hormonal manipulation. In women presenting with proven nodal disease and a tumour unsuitable for wide local excision, chemotherapy is increasingly being given prior to surgery (neo-adjuvant chemotherapy). This has the benefit of demonstrating the efficacy of the chemotherapy, treats systemic disease (which has the greatest impact on long-term survival) and may reduce the size of the primary tumour to such an extent that breast-conserving surgery becomes possible. In a number of women there is a complete clinical and radiological response to chemotherapy, and therefore it is advisable to insert a small titanium clip into the tumour before starting chemotherapy, so that it can be localized when surgery takes place. In patients with extensive co-morbidities that prevent surgery, neo-adjuvant endocrine (primary hormone treatment) can be used.

Surgical: breast surgery is performed to achieve local control of disease, and reduce disease burden to a level that adjuvant treatments can control. In addition, it allows prognostic information to be gained that will guide the choices of subsequent adjuvant treatments. The main choice to be made is between WLE and radiotherapy to the remaining breast, and mastectomy, either of which is combined with axillary lymph node dissection. *These two treatment options offer equivalent long-term survival, and should usually be the choice of the patient.* If there were no pre-operative evidence of axillary nodal spread, then SLN biopsy would be performed at the time of WLE or mastectomy in order to 'stage' the axilla. This procedure avoids much of the morbidity associated with axillary lymph node dissection (seroma, lymphoedema, shoulder pain and stiffness).

Reconstructive surgery should ideally be offered to the patient considering mastectomy, and options include immediate or delayed reconstruction. There are many options available to a woman wanting a breast reconstruction. A reconstructed breast can be formed using implants and tissue expanders alone, endogenous tissues (e.g. latissimus dorsi flap, DIEP flap, TRAM flap etc.) either on their own (autologous) or combined with an implant.

Radiotherapy: there is very good evidence from large randomized controlled trials that radiotherapy reduces local recurrence and improves survival after WLE, making breast-conserving therapy equivalent to mastectomy in terms of long-term survival. Radiotherapy may also be used after mastectomy for large, aggressive tumours with axillary node metastasis, directed towards the chest wall, axilla and supraclavicular fossa.

Chemotherapy: this is offered to women with aggressive tumours in order to reduce the risk of distant metastatic disease. Most women with involved axillary lymph nodes are considered for chemotherapy, women with large, high-grade tumours, or younger women also benefit.

Hormonal manipulation: approximately 70 to 80 per cent of women have oestrogen/progesterone receptor–rich tumours, which makes them sensitive to hormone manipulation. Tamoxifen (a selective estrogen receptor modulator) binds to the oestrogen receptor in breast cells, blocking its action. It is used in pre-menopausal women with oestrogen receptor–positive breast cancer. The Aromatase inhibitor group of drugs prevents androgens from being converted into oestradiol, and is used in post-menopausal women with oestrogen receptor–positive breast cancer. These treatments greatly reduce the risk of breast cancer recurrence, and are generally well tolerated.

Biological therapy: approximately 15 to 20 per cent of breast cancers over-express the epidermal growth factor receptor HER-2/neu, which is an important part of the pathway stimulating tumour growth and preventing cell death. Women with HER-2 positive breast cancers can benefit from treatment with trastuzumab (Herceptin) or similar agents. Trastuzumab is a monoclonal antibody directed against the HER-2 receptor. It is currently given weekly for a year.

ᴨᴨ OSCE Counselling cases

OSCE COUNSELLING CASE 1.11 – 'What can I do about this breast pain?'

Breast pain is surprisingly common amongst women. It may be *cyclical* or *non-cyclical*, and a careful history will determine the timing and any trigger factors. It is important to consider 'non-breast' causes, such as chest wall, neck, back and shoulder pain. After history and examination has excluded any other aetiology, options for managing breast pain can be discussed. Most women will cope with the discomfort once they have been re-assured that there is nothing sinister causing the pain.

The importance of a correctly fitting bra should be emphasized, and specialized sports bras may be useful for periods of vigorous exercise. Reducing caffeine intake, stopping smoking, taking part in regular exercise and reducing dietary fat intake are the most important lifestyle modifications of benefit in women with true breast pain.

Simple analgesics may be appropriate if the pain is only present for a few days during a particular part of the menstrual cycle. Some women find benefit from taking evening primrose oil, which is rich in vitamin E and some essential fatty acids. It needs to be taken at relatively high doses, and for at least 2 months before the peak benefit is obtained, but has relatively few side effects, and can be bought without prescription.

OSCE COUNSELLING CASE 1.12 – 'I'm confused about my surgical options for breast cancer. Which should I choose?'

For most women (except those with very advanced tumours) it has been shown by a number of well-performed studies that breast-conserving therapy (i.e. WLE followed by radiotherapy to the remaining breast) results in the same overall survival rates as mastectomy, and a similarly low rate of local recurrence. Accordingly, the choice of surgery should be the patient's. Whatever approach is used, it should be made clear to the woman that she will be supported with as much information she feels she needs in order to make the decision.

Many women feel that time is critical, and they want to have their operation as soon as possible. It is worth emphasizing that breast cancer is usually very slow growing, and that at the time of diagnosis it may already have been present for many months or even years. Allowing some days, or even a week or two to make a decision will not jeopardize the outcome, but may allow unpressured choices to be made.

Mastectomy has a major impact on the body image of most women. For women who choose mastectomy, or for whom WLE is not appropriate (e.g. previous radiotherapy to that breast, or large or multifocal disease), reconstructive surgery should usually be discussed and offered.

Axillary staging provides prognostic information that influences adjuvant treatment. Sentinel lymph node biopsy is a technique of identifying the first node(s) that drains the breast. This is performed using a dual technique of injected radio-active colloid and blue dye. It has the significant benefit of reduced post-operative morbidity when compared with axillary lymph node dissection. If the sentinel node is clear, the presumption is that the rest of the axillary nodes are also clear. Unfortunately its sensitivity is not 100 per cent, plus if the sentinel node is positive it usually requires further axillary surgery to 'clear' the axilla, or axillary radiotherapy.

REVISION PANEL

- Breast cancer is one of the most common malignancies. The risk of developing breast cancer increases with age.
- Triple assessment – clinical examination, radiological imaging, and cytology and/or histology – underlies the diagnosis of breast lumps. Optimal investigation and treatment is obtained through a multidisciplinary approach.
- Imaging options for the breast include ultrasound, mammography and MRI. Screening mammography programmes are an important means of detecting breast cancer at an earlier point than when clinically apparent, with the hope of improving both individual and population outcomes.
- Surgical treatment of breast cancer continues to evolve, with techniques including breast-conserving treatment, reconstructive and oncoplastic approaches and sentinel node biopsy to minimally assess draining lymph node basins.
- Adjuvant treatment after surgery has an important role in reducing recurrence rates and mortality.

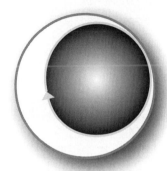

2 Ear, nose and throat (ENT)

Chris Coulson, Adrian Drake-Lee

NOSE: EPISTAXIS

UNILATERAL NASAL DISCHARGE

NASAL OBSTRUCTION

LANGUAGE DELAY AND DEVELOPMENT

ADULT EAR DISEASE

ADULT BILATERAL DEAFNESS

EARACHE

THE DIZZY PATIENT

ACUTE FACIAL PALSY

THROAT

NOSE: EPISTAXIS

Questions

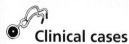

Clinical cases

For each of the clinical case scenarios given

> **Q1:** What is the likely differential diagnosis?
> **Q2:** What additional features in the history would you like to elicit?
> **Q3:** What are the important findings on examination?
> **Q4:** What investigations would be most helpful and why?
> **Q5:** What are the treatment options?

CASE 2.1 – **Adult with nosebleed**

A 60-year-old retired man, who is on warfarin for a deep vein thrombosis (DVT), presents with a profuse epistaxis to the accident and emergency (A&E) department. There is no other significant history. Examination shows that the patient is actively bleeding from the left side of the nose.

CASE 2.2 – **Child with nosebleed**

A 7-year-old girl presents with intermittent bilateral epistaxis to the ENT clinic. Examination of the nose reveals dilated veins anteriorly, but no obvious signs of any other pathology.

👥 OSCE Counselling cases

OSCE COUNSELLING CASE 2.1 – **Adult with nosebleed.**

What advice should you give to an adult male who is coming into hospital and has had his nose packed?

OSCE COUNSELLING CASE 2.2 – **A single mother has a child aged 3 years with profuse intermittent nosebleeds, which occur at night.**

The mother is concerned that her child might bleed to death. Can you assure her that this will not be the case?

Key concepts

- Epistaxis is commonly the result of a localized nasal condition.
- Epistaxis may be caused by a systemic problem.
- Treat the condition locally and then investigate the patient.

Answers

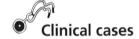 Clinical cases

CASE 2.1 – Adult with nosebleed

A1: What is the likely differential diagnosis?

Epistaxis can be due to a local condition or part of a systemic disease. Most cases are related to dilated vessels on the anterior septum, Little's area, this is the region where the three different vascular supplies to the nose (sphenopalatine artery, ethmoid arteries and facial artery, via the superior labial artery) converge (Figure 2.1). Bleeding from Little's area is especially common in younger adults; it occurs occasionally from the posterior nasal cavity, typically in elderly patients, and is usually related to a recent

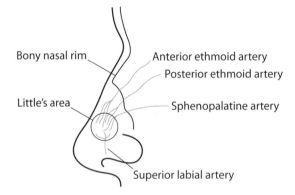

Figure 2.1 Schematic diagram of blood supply to the anterior nose.

upper respiratory tract infection or direct trauma (nose picking). A nasal tumour may present with unilateral epistaxis, although this is not profuse unless it erodes into an artery. The differential diagnosis of systemic diseases causing epistaxis includes any lesion that might interfere with coagulation, including diseases of the bone marrow and liver, and drugs that interact with the clotting cascade.

A2: What additional features in the history would you like to elicit?

Ask about a history of bruising or bleeding elsewhere, as this may indicate a bleeding diathesis. A full general medical history should be taken on any patient who presents with epistaxis once the condition has been treated, with particular reference to diseases (liver dysfunction) or therapies (antiplatelet agents, aspirin or warfarin) that may interfere with clotting.

A3: What are the important findings on examination?

Primary resuscitation measures involve assessing the degree of blood loss and the need for intravenous fluids. Pulse and blood pressure should be checked and aid in determining whether the patient is in shock. The anterior nasal cavity should be examined to determine whether a bleeding point is visible, and if it is, this can be cauterized.

A4: What investigations would be most helpful and why?

Investigations are undertaken after the patient has been assessed and active bleeding stopped if he or she is admitted to hospital. A full blood count (FBC) should be undertaken at the time of bleeding. A clotting screen should be performed to see whether the patient is over-anticoagulated or has a bleeding diathesis.

A5: What are the treatment options?

Priority is to arrest haemorrhage and resuscitate a shocked patient. Initial management follows an escalating scale of interventions, stopping only once the haemorrhage has arrested. Primary management involves squeezing the anterior cartilaginous nose for 10 minutes (Figure 2.2), tamponading the vessels of the anterior septum, with the patient in a head-down, seated position (ensuring ongoing epistaxis does not travel to the nasopharynx and on the pharynx and larynx). This simple measure will stop most nosebleeds. Visual inspection of the anterior nose will permit cauterization of the offending vessels. If this measure fails then nasal packing is required, and this can be performed with a variety of substances, including BIPP (bismuth iodoform paraffin paste) or Merocel packs. Packing the nose is an uncomfortable procedure and should be undertaken under local

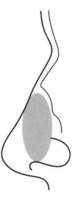

Figure 2.2 Schematic diagram of area of the nose to hold in epistaxis.

anaesthesia (Co-phenylcaine spray – 5 per cent aqueous solution of lignocaine and phenylephrine). If the patient has been over-anticoagulated, correction of this is typically required. If the pack remains in situ over 48 h antibiotic prophylaxis is required because a secondary sinusitis or toxic shock syndrome may develop. All patients with packing should be admitted to the hospital because hypoxia, confusion and inhalation of a pack may occur. Occasionally, operations are required if nasal packing is unsuccessful such as correction of septal displacement so that the nose can be packed very tightly under general anaesthesia or sphenopalatine artery ligation may be undertaken.

CASE 2.2 – **Child with nosebleed**

A1: What is the likely differential diagnosis?

The differential diagnosis is the same as for Case 2.1. However, it is exceptionally rare for systemic disease to present with epistaxis in a child, although acute leukaemia may present in this way. The most common cause is dilated vessels in Little's area where vessels from the internal (anterior and posterior ethmoid arteries) and external (sphenopalatine artery and facial artery) carotid arteries anastomose.

A2: What additional features in the history would you like to elicit?

Additional features in the history are those in Case 2.1. Bruising and other bleeding problems should always be asked about in children with epistaxis. A full history of nasal symptoms such as crusting of the anterior nose should also be taken.

A3: What are the important findings on examination?

Primary resuscitation measures involve assessing the degree of blood loss and the need for intravenous fluids, pulse and blood pressure should be checked and aid in determining whether the patient is in shock, although this is extremely unlikely in a child. The anterior nasal cavity should be examined to determine whether a bleeding point is visible, and if it is, this can be cauterized.

A4: What investigations would be most helpful and why?

Unless systemic disease is suspected, no investigations are required. Occasionally, an FBC is needed if the patient has bled actively and often; however, anaemia is very rare from epistaxis in children.

A5: What are the treatment options?

The treatment in children is slightly different from that in an adult as the cause in a child is often vestibulitis resulting from frequent nose picking. This causes direct trauma to Little's area. A course of Naseptin cream (chlorhexidine hydrochloride and neomycin) to the anterior nasal vestibule on both sides may settle any infection and resolve the condition as the child then picks the nose less frequently. Simple cautery with silver nitrate is effective in over half the cases, and can be undertaken with or without local anaesthesia. If the child is under 5 years old, it is better to perform cautery under general anaesthesia, primarily to keep the child still, to ensure it can be completed effectively. Randomized controlled trials demonstrate an equivalent efficacy for cautery and Naseptin. Parents should be warned that children with epistaxis tend to get further bleeding in half of all cases.

OSCE Counselling cases

OSCE COUNSELLING CASE 2.1 – **What advice should you give to an adult male who is coming into hospital and has had his nose packed?**

The patient should be advised that he will be in hospital between 2 and 3 days. The packing will be in place for 1 to 2 days and may be painful when removed. The patient should also be advised that there might be some fresh bleeding and clots when the packs come out. It is important to stress that a few simple investigations will be done to check the clotting status and this may require treatment as well.

OSCE COUNSELLING CASE 2.2 – **A single mother has a child aged 3 years with profuse intermittent nosebleeds, which occur at night**

It is important to stress that the bleeding always looks a lot worse than the actual amount lost. A simple analogy – that a cup of coffee or a glass of wine looks more when spilt – will often suffice. It is also worthwhile stressing that children often rub the blood on their face while they are having nosebleeds. Counsel the mother that it is perfectly easy to stop most nosebleeds by sitting the child up, asking him to breathe through the mouth and squeezing the cartilaginous part of the nasal septum between the thumb and forefingers for 10 minutes (see Figure 2.2). Treatment can entail cautery or Naseptin cream, although episodes of bleeding that are uncontrollable with conservative measures require cautery to arrest haemorrhage.

REVISION PANEL

- Both adults and children bleed primarily from the anterior septum – Little's area.
- Elderly patients can bleed from the posterior nasal cavity.
- Diagnosis includes identifying the bleeding point and excluding other local and systemic conditions.
- Epistaxis can typically be controlled with squeezing the anterior external nose.
- If epistaxis does not stop with local pressure, nasal cautery is usually effective. Occasionally nasal packing and artery ligation are required to arrest the haemorrhage.

UNILATERAL NASAL DISCHARGE

Questions

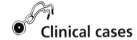

Clinical cases

For each of the clinical case scenarios given

> **Q1:** What is the likely differential diagnosis?
> **Q2:** What additional features in the history would you like to elicit?
> **Q3:** What are the important findings on examination?
> **Q4:** What investigations would be most helpful and why?
> **Q5:** What are the treatment options?

CASE 2.3 – **Child with unilateral discharge**

A child aged 2 years presents with a 1-week history of unilateral nasal discharge.

CASE 2.4 – **Adult with head injury**

A 24-year-old man who had a head injury a month previously with slight concussion has a loss of sense of smell and a unilateral clear discharge from the left side of the nose.

OSCE Counselling cases

OSCE COUNSELLING CASE 2.3 – **The child with unilateral discharge**

How would you counsel the mother of a child who is concerned that the cause of unilateral symptoms could be tumour?

OSCE COUNSELLING CASE 2.4 – **The adult with a cerebrospinal fluid (CSF) leak**

A patient who has had an endo-nasal repair of a cerebrospinal fluid (CSF) leak wonders if there are any particular post-operative instructions.

🔑 Key concepts

- Unilateral mucoid nasal discharge in a child is usually caused by a foreign body.
- Unilateral nasal discharge should be investigated.
- Unilateral clear nasal discharge is CSF until proved otherwise.

Answers

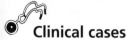
Clinical cases

CASE 2.3 – **Child with unilateral discharge**

A1: What is the likely differential diagnosis?

A foreign body

A2: What additional features in the history would you like to elicit?

Ask the parent if the child put anything into his nose. Remember that other children may have put an object into the child's nose.

A3: What are the important findings on examination?

Examination often reveals unilateral purulent nasal discharge. Depending on the child's age and the cooperation of both child and parent, this can sometimes be suctioned revealing the foreign body. This can often be removed in the outpatient department, although it is critical that you do not cause the child too much distress. If the child is uncooperative, then removal under general anaesthetic should be arranged.

A4: What investigations would be most helpful and why?

No investigations are required for mucoid or purulent discharge. The child should be examined in the operating theatre.

A5: What are the treatment options?

If the foreign body cannot be removed in the outpatient department, the child should be put on the next available operating list and the nose examined under general anaesthesia to exclude a foreign body. The foreign body is usually easily found and removed. The discharge may take a few days to settle, particularly if there is some granulation tissue in the nose. Florid granulations may be removed at the same time. If no foreign body is found the child may have unilateral sinusitis and a washout of the maxillary sinuses can be undertaken at the same time.

CASE 2.4 – **Adult with head injury**

A1: What is the likely differential diagnosis?

The chief worry is a CSF leak. This is the diagnosis of exclusion because sinusitis may occur.

A2: What additional features in the history would you like to elicit?

Ask if there have been any other episodes of discharge before the head injury. If so this changes the probable diagnosis and makes rhinosinusitis more likely. Although spontaneous CSF leaks do occur, they are relatively rare. Ask the standard history for the nose episodes of blockage, running and sneezing. Adults rarely put foreign bodies up their nose unless they have a learning disability or an active psychiatric problem.

A3: What are the important findings on examination?

Anterior rhinoscopy (examination of the anterior nose with a headlight and speculum) and nasal endoscopy occasionally reveal an origin of the CSF leak, a critical feature when planning surgical repair.

A4: What investigations would be most helpful and why?

Collect the fluid to measure Tau protein ($\beta2\beta$-transferrin present in CSF but not nasal secretions). Computed tomography (CT) of the paranasal sinuses and magnetic resonance imaging (MRI) of the anterior cranial fossa should be undertaken. The treatment is simple: the CSF leak should be closed surgically. Treatment with prophylactic antibiotics is controversial and best discussed with a local neurosurgical unit.

A5: What are the treatment options?

Spontaneous cessation of traumatic CSF leaks often occurs within the first 2 weeks. After this period the chance of closure decreases, associated with an increase in the risk of ascending meningitis, and hence surgical closure is recommended. Once the location of the leak has been identified through a combination of endoscopic and CT findings, operative closure can be planned, and this is typically undertaken via an endoscopic nasal approach.

OSCE Counselling cases

OSCE COUNSELLING CASE 2.3 – **The child with unilateral discharge**

Nasal tumours in childhood are extremely rare and tend to present with bleeding or blockage. The common causes of unilateral nasal blockage are foreign body or sinusitis. It is therefore possible to be reassuring. Additionally, once the patient has been examined, a foreign body can be quickly determined and treated.

OSCE COUNSELLING CASE 2.4 – **The adult with a CSF leak**

The patient needs to avoid any preventable rises in CSF pressure as this may displace the repair causing the leak to recommence. Hence, if the patient needs to sneeze, he or she is advised to do this with his or her mouth open (and hand covering this); the patient should avoid straining during defecation and in some cases this may entail prescribing laxatives. Patients should not lift heavy objects for a minimum of a week.

REVISION PANEL

- Unilateral nasal discharge always indicates an underlying pathology; the age of the patient often predicts the cause.
- Children are likely to have a foreign body causing unilateral discharge, and examination under anaesthesia is needed if an obvious cause cannot be seen in clinic.
- Clinicians should have a high index of suspicion of a CSF leak if a patient presents with a clear nasal discharge post head injury.
- The diagnosis of a CSF leak requires confirmation of CSF (Tau protein) and localization of the leak (endoscopic examination + CT ± MRI).

NASAL OBSTRUCTION

Questions

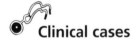

Clinical cases

For each of the clinical case scenarios given

Q1: What is the likely differential diagnosis?
Q2: What additional features in the history would you like to elicit?
Q3: What should one look for in the examination?
Q4: What investigations would be most helpful and why?
Q5: What are the treatment options?

CASE 2.5 – **Child with nasal obstruction and snoring**

A child aged 7 presents with blocked nose and snoring at night. The mother asks that the adenoids be removed to improve the symptoms.

CASE 2.6 – **Adolescent with nasal trauma**

A 17-year-old teenager had trauma to his nose 6 months previously and comes to the clinic with his father. He requests surgery to sort out his nasal obstruction.

👥 OSCE Counselling cases

OSCE COUNSELLING CASE 2.5 – **A mother asks whether their cat should be removed if this causes allergic rhinitis**

OSCE COUNSELLING CASE 2.6 – **What advice should you give to a boy who wants to continue playing football and judo when he has repeated injuries to his nose?**

🔑 Key concepts

- Bilateral nasal discharge is often the result of allergy rather than an adenoid problem.
- Treat allergy medically.
- Treat septal deformity by surgery when contact sport has ceased.

Answers

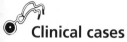
Clinical cases

CASE 2.5 – **Child with nasal obstruction and snoring**

A1: What is the likely differential diagnosis?

Rhinitis, commonly allergic, or physical obstruction due to adenoid hypertrophy

A2: What additional features in the history would you like to elicit?

Determine whether the nasal obstruction fluctuates from side to side and whether it is seasonal or continuous. Seasonal symptoms and fluctuating symptoms are more likely to be allergic in origin. Continuous symptoms are either due to a perennial allergy (house dust mites or pets) or enlarged adenoids. Ask whether obstructive apnoea is present at night, as this is much more common in children aged under 4 years. Other nasal symptoms include sneezing attacks, or clear or mucoid running nasal discharge. Older children and adults may complain of postnasal drip, changes in the sense of smell and facial pain. Asthma and rhinitis often coexist.

A3: What should one look for in the examination?

Watch the child in the clinic. If a child is breathing through his or her nose, the adenoids cannot be hypertrophied. Adenoid hypertrophy causes permanent nasal obstruction and these children sit with their mouths open. It is important to examine the tonsils because large tonsils may cause mouth breathing. The tip of a child's nose turns up easily to help when looking at the mucosa. A purple colour suggests allergy. Place a metal spatula under the nose and observe the misting pattern to ensure both nasal cavities are patent.

A4: What investigations would be most helpful and why?

Undertake allergy testing if history and examination suggest rhinitis.

A5: What are the treatment options?

If the child has an obvious allergic rhinitis, confirmed on skin prick testing, the standard treatment is avoidance of the allergen, if at all possible, followed by medical treatment. Surgery has little part to play. If there is no sign of rhinitis then adenoidal hypertrophy is likely, and these may be removed surgically. The risks of surgery should not be underestimated and primarily involve bleeding. This may occur immediately or 10 days post-operatively. The patient and parents should be warned about a change in voice after the nasal blockage has resolved.

CASE 2.6 – **Adolescent with nasal trauma**

A1: What is the likely differential diagnosis?

Nasal trauma leading to nasal and septal deviation

A2: What additional features in the history would you like to elicit?

Take the same history as for Case 2.5, but always ask about contact sport.

A3: What should one look for in the examination?

Examine the bony pyramid of the nose and make sure that this has not been fractured – this is best performed by looking at the seated patient from behind and noting any nasal deviation. Look at the cartilaginous septum to see whether this is displaced at either side. Turn the tip of the nose up to see whether the front part of the septum has been dislocated outwards.

A4: What investigations would be most helpful and why?

Undertake allergy testing on all patients who have bilateral nasal obstruction because many will have an allergic rhinitis. It is rarely necessary to undertake any other investigations.

A5: What are the treatment options?

Do not advise nasal surgery except for manipulation of a fracture when the risk of re-injury is high. Surgery should not be undertaken until 18 years of age because the nose is still growing and surgery may adversely affect the growth plates. Avoid septal surgery if the child plays a contact sport.

OSCE Counselling cases

OSCE COUNSELLING CASE 2.5 – **A mother asks whether their cat should be removed if this causes allergic rhinitis**

Frequently children are not concerned about their nasal symptoms but the parents are. The cat may be more important to the child than the symptoms. Cats should be excluded from bedrooms. If the child is severely disturbed by the symptoms it may be necessary to re-house a pet. A cat must go if it causes severe asthma.

OSCE COUNSELLING CASE 2.6 – **What advice should you give to a boy who wants to continue playing football and judo when he has repeated injuries to his nose?**

Stress that surgery on the septum makes the structure weaker and more prone to further damage. Should another injury occur cosmetic deformity could be extreme and exceptionally difficult to correct. The septum can be corrected at any time, because nasal obstruction is not a life-threatening condition.

REVISION PANEL

- Full rhinological history and examination are always necessary as allergy often co-exists with other rhinological complaints and needs treating.
- Childhood non-traumatic nasal blockage is typically due to allergy or enlarged adenoids.
- Allergic rhinitis is treated with allergen avoidance and, if unsuccessful, medical therapy.
- Septal surgery is not advised in childhood and should be delayed until after 18 years of age.

LANGUAGE DELAY AND DEVELOPMENT

Questions

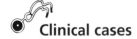 **Clinical cases**

For each of the clinical case scenarios given

Q1: What is the likely differential diagnosis?
Q2: What additional features in the history would you like to elicit?
Q3: What should one look for in the examination?
Q4: What investigations would be most helpful and why?
Q5: What are the treatment options?

CASE 2.7 – **Parents are worried about a 1-year-old who is not speaking**

CASE 2.8 – **A mother comes with a child of three and a half who is badly behaved and also not talking well**

♟♟ OSCE Counselling cases

OSCE COUNSELLING CASE 2.7 – **Parents would like their 3-year-old child's hearing tested, but would like you to explain how this is possible**

OSCE COUNSELLING CASE 2.8 – **What advice would you give to a mother who is concerned about swimming and grommets?**

Key concepts

- Language delay may be the result of hearing loss, which may be sensorineural or conductive. Sensorineural hearing loss is reduction in cochlea or cochlear nerve function. In children this is typically congenital, due to genetic defects, syndrome or intrauterine infections, or acquired secondary to birth trauma or infections like meningitis (Figure 2.3).
- Conductive hearing loss is the reduction of the external and/or middle ear's ability to conduct sound into the inner ear (cochlea). In children it is often associated with normal cochlea function – no associated sensorineural hearing loss.
- Assess development.

- Genetic 50 per cent – Typically related to dysplasia of the cochlea
  - Syndromic 20 per cent
    - Autosomal recessive
      - *Pendred's syndrome* – SNHL and a thyroid goitre
      - *Usher's syndrome* – SNHL and retinitis pigmentosa
      - Revel and Lange-Neilson – prolonged Q-T and SNHL
    - Autosomal dominant
      - *Waardenburg's syndrome* – telecanthus, pigment disorders and SNHL
      - *Treacher Collins syndrome* – hypoplasia of the malar bones, maxilla and mandible; there may be microtia or multiple, external and inner ear abnormalities
    - X-linked
      - Mitochondrial
      - Chromosomal
  - Nonsyndromic 80 per cent
    - Autosomal recessive 80 per cent – Connexin 26
    - Autosomal dominant 20 per cent
    - X-linked
    - Mitochondrial
    - Chromosomal
- Acquired 50 per cent
  - Prenatal
    - Non-infective insults – environmental hazards, diabetes, toxaemia, ototoxic drugs, teratogens (alcohol)
    - Infections – rubella, cytomegalovirus (CMV), measles, chickenpox, herpes, toxoplasmosis, syphilis, HIV
    - It has been suggested that up to 30 per cent of all childhood sensorineural deafness is due to CMV, the onset of which is delayed in 40 to 50 per cent.
    - Risk of congenital hearing loss following maternal rubella is 50 per cent. The classic congenital rubella syndrome (CRS) comprises a triad of hearing loss, cataracts, cardiac abnormalities
  - Perinatal
    - Hypoxia
    - Hyperbilirubinaemia
    - Low birth weight
    - Jaundice
  - Postnatal
    - Infections
      - Acute/chronic otitis media and complications
      - Meningitis – most common cause of acquired sensorineural hearing loss in children
      - Viral labyrinthitis including measles and mumps
      - AIDS
      - Ototoxic drugs
      - Trauma – temporal bone fractures
      - Neoplasia
      - Developmental – delayed auditory maturation
  - Genetic causes – those that present later – Pendred's, large vestibular aqueducts

Figure 2.3 Causes of congenital sensorineural hearing loss.

- Treat mild to severe bilateral sensorineural hearing loss with a hearing aid.
- Treat bilateral profound hearing loss by cochlear implantation.
- Children may swim with grommets in situ.

Answers

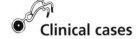

Clinical cases

CASE 2.7 – **Parents are worried about a 1-year-old who is not speaking**

A1: What is the likely differential diagnosis?

Variation in speech development is common, typically investigations start for children who do not speak between 18 months and 2 years, unless there are risk factors (see A2).

A2: What additional features in the history would you like to elicit?

Determine whether the child is at risk of developing sensorineural hearing loss. Risks include prematurity, jaundice, hypoxia or a difficult birth, infections either during pregnancy or postpartum (e.g. measles or rubella), neonatal unit admission and a family history of hearing loss. Ask whether the child babbled and responded to sound when younger. Also ask about the developmental milestones during the first year, and the age of sitting, crawling and use of a spoon. Sometimes language delay is the result of a general developmental delay, so is it important to exclude this.

A3: What should one look for in the examination?

Observe the child while he is sitting in the clinic and see whether he responds to sound when people move around behind him. Examine the ears and determine whether there is a congenital deformity (altered position or shape), increasing the risk of a syndrome with hearing loss. Make sure that both the eardrums and middle ears are normal and that there is no glue ear (otitis media with effusion).

A4: What investigations would be most helpful and why?

See explanation of hearing tests in OSCE answer. This child is too young for subjective audiometry and hence objective audiometry is required. A tympanogram may demonstrate an effusion (glue ear). Otoacoustic emissions testing can demonstrate whether the cochlea outer hair cells are functioning. Hearing thresholds are determined by evoked response audiometry. Depending on whether sensorineural hearing loss is confirmed, further investigations to determine potential congenital causes are undertaken (Figure 2.3).

A5: What are the treatment options?

This depends on the underlying cause. If the child does have bilateral sensorineural hearing loss, it is important to provide hearing aids so that language development can occur as quickly as possible. If the child has a profound sensorineural hearing loss, or does not improve with hearing aids, a cochlear implant should be considered. The earlier a cochlear implant is inserted the better the long-term result. If surgery is undertaken before the age of 2 years, the child stands a very good chance of developing normal language. If the child has glue ear that does not resolve after 3 months of observation, it can be treated with ventilation tubes (grommets) or hearing aids.

CASE 2.8 – **A mother comes with a child of three and a half who is badly behaved and also not talking well**

A1: What is the likely differential diagnosis?

Otitis media with effusion – glue ear

A2: What additional features in the history would you like to elicit?

Ask whether language development was normal previously or whether this change in behaviour and language has suddenly happened. Determine if the child has any older brothers and sisters, because language may be slower in later children. Exclude recurrent acute otitis media (episodes of pain and hearing loss) and discharging ears in a child of this age. There may occasionally be a sensorineural hearing loss, particularly if the child has had meningitis, so a full past history should be taken. However, the most likely cause at this age is glue ear (otitis media with effusion).

A3: What should one look for in the examination?

The patient requires examination of the ears, nose and throat.

Ear: inspection of the pinna and outer ear canal (any congenital deformities which are often linked with middle-ear pathology, perforated acute otitis media will reveal pus in the external canal)

Otoscopy: examine the ear canal looking for discharge and patency. Inspect the tympanic membrane and determine whether it is intact, perforated or if a cholesteatoma is present. The middle ear can be examined through the tympanic membrane – in acute otitis media the ear is bulging with (yellow) pus behind the drum. In glue ear there is no bulging, but a straw-coloured fluid behind the drum, often with bubbles in the middle ear.

Nasal patency should be examined by seeing if a metal spatula placed under the nares (nostrils) mists bilaterally.

The neck should be examined for masses, especially thyroid and branchial cysts – associated with features in Pendred's syndrome and branchial otorenal syndrome.

A4: What investigations would be most helpful and why?

Children of this age may be old enough to undertake a pure-tone audiogram but may require conditioned response audiometry – see OSCE case on audiometry. Tympanometry can determine whether glue ear is present.

A5: What are the treatment options?

A child with glue ear and language delay should have ventilation tubes (grommets) inserted, although hearing aids are another option. Behavioural problems reinforce the need to intervene. It is normal practice to observe the condition to see whether the glue ear resolves over a 3-month period. As many of these children have been seen at least 2 or 3 months before their ENT clinic visit the effusion is usually previously documented.

OSCE Counselling cases

OSCE COUNSELLING CASE 2.7 – Parents would like their 3-year-old child's hearing tested, but would like you to explain how this is possible

Audiological testing can be broadly split into subjective and objective testing. Subjective testing requires active input from the patient to inform the tester of the sounds he/she can hear. Pure tone audiometry is the commonest subjective test, sounds are presented to each ear in turn by headphones and the patient presses a button when he or she can hear the tone (air conduction). A range of tones are tested in each ear. A bone conducting device is then used to determine the cochlea function (due to bone conduction directly stimulating the cochlea, bypassing the outer and middle ear) using a similar process. Children can be conditioned to perform a task when they hear a sound (put a toy in a boat etc.) rather than press a button.

Objective testing does not require patient input and hence can be used at all ages. Evoked response audiometry involves interpreting electrical activity in the brain in response to sound presented by headphones. When the patient's brain detects a sound, there is a change in response demonstrating the threshold of hearing. Tympanometry involves measuring the reflection of sound off the eardrum whilst the pressure in the external ear is altered. This can determine whether there is fluid in the middle ear (glue ear or acute otitis media) or air at normal pressure as occurs in a normal middle ear. Otoacoustic emissions test the function of the outer hair cells in the cochlea. These are typically damaged in sensorineural hearing loss. Normal outer hair cells create a sound in response to detecting sound. This can be detected determining whether the hair cells are functioning normally.

OSCE COUNSELLING CASE 2.8 – What advice would you give to a mother who is concerned about swimming and grommets?

There is much controversy about swimming and grommets. Work from Australia would suggest that the prevalence of discharge is no greater in children who swim with grommets than in those who do not. A child should not dive or jump into water. Hair washing is more risky because the soap or detergent reduces the surface tension and makes middle-ear contamination and discharge more likely. Advise parents to protect the ears in younger children and ask the child to make sure that water and soap do not run into the ear during a shower or bath.

REVISION PANEL

- Assessment of a child with hearing loss requires the assessment of risk factors for sensorineural hearing loss and global development.
- Audiological testing can differentiate sensorineural and conductive hearing losses.
- A child with severe to profound sensorineural hearing loss requires fitting of hearing aids as soon as possible followed by assessment for cochlear implantation.
- Conductive hearing losses are commonly caused by glue ear and can be treated with ventilation tubes (grommets) or hearing aids.

ADULT EAR DISEASE

Questions

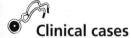
Clinical cases

For each of the clinical case scenarios given

> **Q1:** What is the likely differential diagnosis?
> **Q2:** What additional features in the history would you like to elicit?
> **Q3:** What is the important finding on examination?
> **Q4:** What investigations would be most helpful and why?
> **Q5:** What are the treatment options?

CASE 2.9 – **Ear discharge**

A 25-year-old man presents with progressive hearing loss of 3 years and recently an intermittent, but scanty, smelly discharge.

CASE 2.10 – **Progressive hearing loss**

A woman aged 53 years presents with a 12-month history of a progressive, left-sided, sensorineural hearing loss with occasional tinnitus.

OSCE Counselling cases

OSCE COUNSELLING CASE 2.9 – **What advice would you give to the patient who is having a mastoid exploration?**

OSCE COUNSELLING CASE 2.10 – **A patient with a unilateral acoustic neuroma wants to know the risk of developing one on the other side. What is your advice to the patient?**

Key concepts

- Unilateral discharge with mucus means that there is a tympanic membrane perforation.
- Unilateral discharge which smells foul suggests a cholesteatoma.
- Always examine the eardrum.
- A unilateral sensorineural hearing loss needs MRI to exclude an acoustic neuroma.

Answers

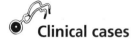

Clinical cases

CASE 2.9 – **Ear discharge**

A1: What is the likely differential diagnosis?

The differential diagnosis includes otitis externa, or chronic middle-ear disease (chronic otitis media), either a perforation or a cholesteatoma. A carcinoma is very rare.

A2: What additional features in the history would you like to elicit?

Ask about any hearing loss, pain, discharge, dizziness and tinnitus for each ear. Ask about the relationships between the symptoms. If a patient has a progressive hearing loss together with an intermittent scanty discharge, but no pain, it suggests a chronic middle-ear problem. If there is pain the patient may have had either an acute middle-ear infection (acute otitis media) or otitis externa. If the discharge is profuse and mucoid, it comes from the middle ear, so the eardrum must be perforated. (There are mucus glands in the middle ear, but not in the external ear.) Middle-ear disease may produce vertigo but the dizzy patient is considered later and you are referred to Cases 2.13 and 2.14.

A3: What is the important finding on examination?

The external ear canal and drum should be inspected. Start with the better ear and then proceed to the diseased side. Note whether there is any wax or debris in the external canal. This requires removal because the eardrum must be inspected fully. Do not syringe a discharging ear as this may transmit infection medially. The history in this case suggests chronic middle-ear disease with cholesteatoma. Cholesteatoma is the presence of squamous epithelium in the middle ear. This is thought to arise as a repercussion of ear infections. It can erode into middle-ear structures (ossicles, labyrinth, facial nerve) and may give rise to intracranial complications; this is why it is important to diagnose the condition. Brown/white smelly discharge is seen in the attic and also sometimes in the posterior part of the eardrum.

A4: What investigations would be most helpful and why?

This patient should have a pure-tone audiogram. High-resolution computed tomography (HRCT) of the temporal bone is performed and can demonstrate the extent of disease and the presence of complications – erosion of the semicircular canals, facial canals or tegmen tympani.

A5: What are the treatment options?

If a cholesteatoma is present, mastoid surgery is required to remove the disease and prevent intracranial or intratemporal complications. If the patient has an infected perforation, this is initially treated with antibiotic eardrops and a tympanoplasty (repair of eardrum with or without ossicle reconstruction) can be considered.

CASE 2.10 – **Progressive hearing loss**

A1: What is the likely differential diagnosis?

Typically a unilateral, progressive, sensorineural hearing loss has no identifiable cause, an acoustic neuroma must be excluded (i.e. a tumour of the eighth nerve, which usually arises in the internal acoustic meatus and can extend into the intracranial cavity by the brain stem). Occasionally, a unilateral sensorineural hearing loss may arise from a viral infection or ischaemia, particularly in older patients.

A2: What additional features in the history would you like to elicit?

Ask about any hearing loss, pain, discharge, dizziness and tinnitus for each ear. Large acoustic neuromas can cause facial nerve, trigeminal nerve and bulbar nerve dysfunction.

A3: What is the important finding on examination?

The external ear canal and drum should be inspected. Start with the better ear and then proceed to the diseased side. Note whether there is any wax or debris in the external canal. This requires removal because the eardrum must be inspected fully. A patient with a sensorineural hearing loss with no other obvious cause has a normal eardrum. Tuning fork tests would demonstrate a Weber lateralizing to the better hearing ear in a sensorineural hearing loss.

Cranial nerves should be examined and an assessment of balance function undertaken – heal-toe gait. Patients with presbycusis typically have otoscopically normal ears.

A4: What investigations would be most helpful and why?

The patient should have an audiogram to determine whether the loss is conductive or sensorineural. If sensorineural is confirmed, then an MRI scan is arranged to exclude a cerebellopontine angle lesion, typically an acoustic neuroma, causing the loss.

A5: What are the treatment options?

The majority of patients investigated for unilateral or asymmetric sensorineural hearing loss have no underlying cause found. Approximately 1.5 per cent have an acoustic neuroma causing their symptoms; this is a benign tumour of Schwann cells of, usually, the vestibular nerve. Two-thirds of acoustic neuromas do not grow in the long term. The primary management strategy for <2-cm tumours is conservative with a wait-and-rescan policy. The patient is scanned at increasing intervals to confirm it is static. If the tumour grows then it can be treated with stereotactic radiosurgery or surgical excision.

Rehabilitation of the patient's hearing can be performed with a conventional hearing aid, or bone-anchored hearing aid.

OSCE Counselling cases

OSCE COUNSELLING CASE 2.9 – What advice would you give to the patient who is having a mastoid exploration?

The aims of mastoid surgery are twofold, to prevent potential intracranial and intratemporal complications of a cholesteatoma (these are thankfully rare and occur in 4 per cent per decade the disease is present), and to improve symptoms – chiefly discharge and malodour, but also potential hearing loss although hearing may be worse after surgery. There is a very small risk to the facial nerve while undertaking middle-ear surgery, although the chance of damage is similar to the chance of disease-related facial palsy if no surgery is undertaken. The disease may require some form of follow-up for life if a mastoid cavity is created during surgery. Surgery often removes the self-cleansing external ear skin and so wax and debris accumulate.

OSCE COUNSELLING CASE 2.10 – A patient with a unilateral acoustic neuroma wants to know the risk of developing one on the other side. What is your advice to the patient?

Unless a patient has neurofibromatosis type 2, the risk of developing bilateral acoustic neuroma is incredibly rare. It is possible to hear with one ear perfectly satisfactorily. Problems may occur in localizing sound and discrimination in a noisy environment.

REVISION PANEL

- A discharging ear is always pathological; the clinician should examine the ear thoroughly to determine the cause.
- Copious mucoid discharge is from a middle-ear infection with a perforated tympanic membrane.
- Scanty discharge is due to a cholesteatoma or otitis externa – the diagnosis is made on examination.
- A unilateral sensorineural hearing loss is typically idiopathic; however, it may be caused by an acoustic neuroma.

ADULT BILATERAL DEAFNESS

Questions

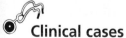
Clinical cases

For the clinical case scenario given

> **Q1:** What is the likely differential diagnosis?
> **Q2:** What additional features in the history would you like to elicit?
> **Q3:** What is the important finding on examination?
> **Q4:** What investigations would be most helpful and why?
> **Q5:** What are the treatment options?

CASE 2.11 – **Adult with bilateral deafness**

A 66-year-old man comes to the department with decreased hearing over the previous 7 years and both ears are the same.

♟ OSCE Counselling case

OSCE COUNSELLING CASE 2.11 – **A patient wants to use a hearing aid but feels that it will exacerbate the condition. What is your advice?**

Key concepts

- Presbycusis (age-related hearing loss) may require a hearing aid.
- Hearing aids work if the patient requests them.

Answers

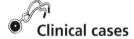

Clinical cases

CASE 2.11 – **Adult with bilateral deafness**

A1: What is the likely differential diagnosis?

Presbycusis

A2: What additional features in the history would you like to elicit?

Ask about any hearing loss, pain, discharge, dizziness and tinnitus for each ear. Ask about risk factors for hearing loss/ear disease:

- Ear operations – may have iatrogenic cause of hearing loss
- Ear infections – can cause conductive or sensorineural hearing loss, or represent chronic otitis media
- Noise exposure – occupational history
- Head injuries – ask an occupational history
- Systemic diseases such as diabetes mellitus and cardiovascular atheroma may exacerbate the ageing changes
- Previous/current use of ototoxic medications
- Family history of hearing loss

Ask whether the patient wants a hearing aid – relatives often want the device rather than the patient. This is a recipe for failure.

A3: What is the important finding on examination?

Patients with presbycusis typically have otoscopically normal ears.

A4: What investigations would be most helpful and why?

Assess the degree of hearing loss in both the low and the high frequencies. The high-frequency component is the element associated with articulation. Patients will often say that they hear what people say but they cannot understand.

A5: What are the treatment options?

Most patients who have a moderate hearing loss or greater require a hearing aid but the patient has to accept this before it is worth prescribing one. If a patient is in two minds one should be tried for a period and returned if it is unsatisfactory. Further audiometric assessment may be undertaken after a year if a patient is unhappy with the hearing aid.

OSCE Counselling case

OSCE COUNSELLING CASE 2.11 – **A patient wants to use a hearing aid but feels that it will exacerbate the condition. What is your advice?**

There is no evidence that wearing a hearing aid worsens any sensorineural hearing loss. Stress that the hearing will change over time and become slightly worse irrespective of whether or not a hearing aid is used.

REVISION PANEL

- Bilateral sensorineural hearing loss is a common finding in the elderly.
- Diagnosis of presbycusis requires exclusion of other otological conditions and the audiometric confirmation of symmetrical sensorineural hearing loss, worse in the high frequencies.
- Treatment of presbycusis involves reassurance that there is not a sinister cause and discussions regarding the patient's desire to wear a hearing aid.

EARACHE

Questions

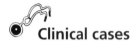

Clinical cases

For each of the clinical case scenarios given

> **Q1:** What is the likely differential diagnosis?
> **Q2:** What additional features in the history would you like to elicit?
> **Q3:** What is the important finding on examination?
> **Q4:** What investigations would be most helpful and why?
> **Q5:** What are the treatment options?

CASE 2.12 – **Child with earache**

A child aged 3 years has an acute earache, which has started that day.

CASE 2.13 – **Adult with earache**

An adult aged 37 years presents with intermittently painful ears, mostly affecting the right side.

OSCE Counselling case

OSCE COUNSELLING CASE 2.12 – **A patient wants to swim when you have diagnosed otitis externa. What is your advice?**

🔑 Key concepts

- Acute otitis media may be treated conservatively, if mild.
- Do not poke the ears in otitis externa.
- Pain may be referred to the ears from the jaw or the neck.

Answers

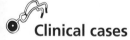 **Clinical cases**

CASE 2.12 – **Child with earache**

A1: What is the likely differential diagnosis?

The most likely diagnosis is acute otitis media. Other structures may refer pain to the ear and a teething child may have pain, which can be difficult to distinguish from a middle-ear problem.

A2: What additional features in the history would you like to elicit?

Ask if the child has a respiratory infection. How severe is the pain? This can be gauged by asking whether the child is kept awake at night, holds his ear and wants to go to bed. Ascertain the relationship between pain, hearing loss and discharge. Patients with pain, hearing loss and no discharge have acute otitis media. If discharge starts and the pain and hearing loss resolve, this is due to the tympanic membrane perforating reducing the pressure in the middle ear.

A3: What is the important finding on examination?

Examine both ears and see whether one sticks out more than the other. In acute mastoiditis, a complication of acute otitis media, there is often a swelling behind the ear and it is pushed forwards and slightly downwards. Examine the better ear first. Children often have a pink eardrum when they have a cold. If both ears look the same, acute otitis media is unlikely. If there is pus behind the drum (diagnostic of acute otitis media), it looks yellow and bulging. This is most obvious in the posterosuperior region and this is the most common site of rupture. If the eardrum has not been examined, the diagnosis of acute otitis media is presumptive.

A4: What investigations would be most helpful and why?

No investigations are required for simple acute otitis media.

A5: What are the treatment options?

There is much debate about the need for antibiotic chemotherapy in acute otitis media. There have been many obvious flaws in the clinical trials conducted in this area. Basically, if the child is well and has little in the way of constitutional symptoms, no treatment is required. If the child has mild discomfort, treat with analgesia, because the condition will settle in the vast majority of cases. If the child is unwell and the eardrum is bulging dramatically, treat with antibiotics such as amoxicillin at the appropriate dose for the weight and age of the child. If the child is vomiting, the first dose should be given intramuscularly. Erythromycin is a suitable alternative if the child is sensitive to penicillin. Very occasionally intracranial sepsis follows acute ear infections.

CASE 2.13 – **Adult with earache**

A1: What is the likely differential diagnosis?

The most likely causes of earache in the adult are either otitis externa or referred otalgia. Young adults may have temporomandibular problems and questions about chewing and pain will help to determine if this is the cause. Elderly people may have problems with the cervical spine, which also causes a referred otalgia. Otitis externa may go from ear to ear and there is a period of irritation followed by self-inflicted trauma and secondary infection. The cycle repeats itself.

A2: What additional features in the history would you like to elicit?

Ascertain the relationship between pain, discharge and hearing loss. In acute otitis externa, there is typically scanty discharge, severe pain, but no hearing loss. There is usually a precipitating history of trauma, cotton buds or water exposure, swimming or syringing. Patients with acute otitis media also often complain of itching.

A3: What is the important finding on examination?

Examine the better ear first so that it can be compared with the one causing the problem. If there is debris, this should be removed. The diagnosis of otitis externa cannot be made until the drum has been examined and is shown to be intact. Sometimes there is a secondary otitis externa when there is a perforation, but mucus means that there is middle-ear disease. There are three common types of otitis externa: a furuncle in the hair-bearing area, and diffuse oedematous and diffuse eczematous otitis externa. Examine the temporomandibular joint and neck. Some patients poke their ears if there is pain there and set up secondary otitis externa.

A4: What investigations would be most helpful and why?

No investigations are mandatory, although an ear swab may help with antibiotic sensitivity. The infecting organism is *Pseudomonas aeruginosa* in most cases.

A5: What are the treatment options?

Treatment is meticulous aural toilet. Once the debris is removed, treat with antibiotic eardrops. Tell the patient to keep the ear dry and not to poke it. If the problem does not settle easily, referral to the ENT department may be required. Patients with diabetes mellitus need careful monitoring because they may develop a severe otitis externa called malignant otitis externa. The condition may erode into the cranial cavity and can be fatal.

ᴦᴦ OSCE Counselling case

OSCE COUNSELLING CASE 2.12 – **A patient wants to swim when you have diagnosed otitis externa. What is your advice?**

No. The patient should be symptom free for 3 months before re-commencing swimming.

REVISION PANEL

- Acute otitis media is generally a self-limiting infection treated initially with conservative therapy.
- If there is no resolution of acute otitis media after 48 hours, antibiotic therapy is commenced.
- Mastoiditis and intracranial sepsis are rare complications of acute otitis media.
- Acute otitis externa typically presents after trauma, direct or water, to the ear canal.
- Treatment of acute otitis externa is with aural toilet and antibiotic drops.

THE DIZZY PATIENT

Questions

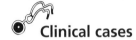 **Clinical cases**

For the clinical case scenario given

> **Q1:** What is the likely differential diagnosis?
> **Q2:** What additional features in the history would you like to elicit?
> **Q3:** What should one look for in the examination?
> **Q4:** What investigations would be most helpful and why?
> **Q5:** What are the treatment options?

CASE 2.14 – **Dizziness**

An adult presents with dizziness when she turns her head and rolls over in bed. She says that it comes from the left side of the head.

OSCE Counselling case

OSCE COUNSELLING CASE 2.13 – **The patient is obviously worried that there is something sinister going on. What is your advice?**

🔑 Key concepts

- Dizziness may be unsteadiness or true vertigo.
- True vertigo coming from the labyrinth never causes unconsciousness.
- Vertigo on head movements for a few seconds is benign positional vertigo.
- Episodic vertigo with hearing loss and tinnitus may be Ménière's disease.

Answers

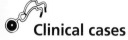 **Clinical cases**

CASE 2.14 – **Dizziness**

A1: What is the likely differential diagnosis?

- Benign positional vertigo
- Ménière's disease
- Vestibular neuronitis/labyrinthitis

A2: What additional features in the history would you like to elicit?

Determine whether the patient has true vertigo, rather than unsteadiness. Vertigo is the hallucination of movement; either the environment moves or the patient moves. Ask the patient whether she has had similar attacks before and whether the attacks are episodic. Ask how long each attack is. If it is for a few seconds without hearing loss and tinnitus, it is likely to be benign positional vertigo. Ménière's disease tends to present with tinnitus and hearing loss, together with the vertigo, over a period of hours. Vestibular neuronitis lasts for days and will not be associated with other ear symptoms. Ask about unconsciousness. Patients with peripheral lesions are conscious whereas those with central nervous system problems, which may be vascular in origin, can lose consciousness. Ask whether epileptic attacks occur. A full general history should be taken for all patients with dizziness, including cardiovascular, respiratory, central nervous and gastrointestinal symptoms. Many patients with vascular disease and hypertension feel unsteady when they stand up.

Investigations include audiometry and occasionally caloric testing if there is any diagnostic doubt. If the diagnosis is benign positional vertigo, no further investigation is required. If there is asymmetrical hearing, MRI of the internal auditory meatus should be arranged.

A3: What should one look for in the examination?

A full otoneurological examination should be undertaken; this includes examination of the ears, plus tests to exclude central pathology – examination of the cranial nerves, pursuit and tests for cerebellar signs. Pulse and blood pressure should be measured. If a patient has good mobility of the cervical spine, positional tests should be undertaken. The most likely diagnosis here is benign positional paroxysmal vertigo. This is confirmed by Dix-Hallpike testing – lying the patient down from a seated position with the patient's head rotated 30 degrees to the affected side. The patient develops geotropic rotational nystagmus with an additional downbeat component (Figure 2.4). If the patient has cervical spine problems then a Dix-Hallpike is contraindicated.

A4: What investigations would be most helpful and why?

An audiogram should be performed. If benign positional paroxysmal vertigo (BPPV) is confirmed on Dix-Hallpike testing, then no further investigations are required.

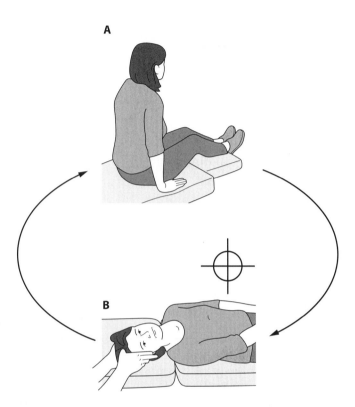

Figure 2.4 Dix-Hallpike test for benign positional paroxysmal vertigo.

A5: What are the treatment options?

Treatment for benign positional vertigo is to perform a particle repositioning manoeuvre (the Epley manoeuvre) (Figure 2.5), although often the symptoms settle spontaneously. Ménière's disease is typically treated in a stepwise manner, commencing with conservative measures – low-salt diet, caffeine and alcohol avoidance – which are successful in controlling symptoms in 60 per cent of patients. In those who fail conservative measures, medical therapy with Betahistine (a histamine analogue which effects microcirculation within the cochlea and vestibular system) is attempted, again this is successful in approximately 60 per cent of patients. Finally destruction of the labyrinth, either chemically with gentamycin or surgically, stops almost all attacks of Ménière's, although patients may develop a chronic imbalance due to unilateral labyrinthine failure. Vestibular neuronitis presents with a picture identical to unilateral vestibular loss and can be treated with vestibular therapy.

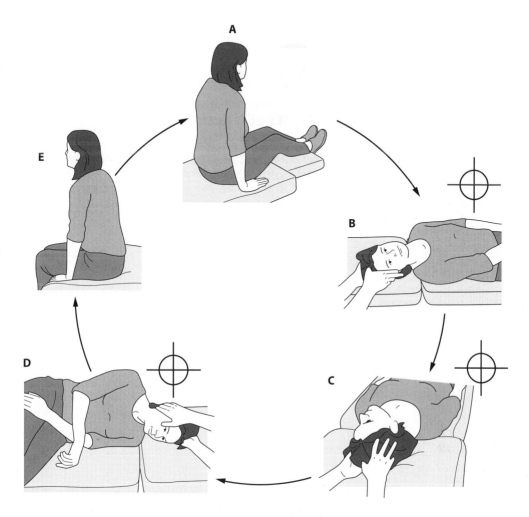

Figure 2.5 Epley manoeuvre for benign positional paroxysmal vertigo.

👥 OSCE Counselling case

OSCE COUNSELLING CASE 2.13 – **The patient is obviously worried that there is something sinister going on. What is your advice?**

As it is very easy to make the diagnosis, you can inform the patient that the disease is coming from the inner ear and that he does not have a serious brain condition. Patients are often worried about this and they may not volunteer the information, so mention it. State that the condition is often self-limiting but relapses in 50 per cent and a further Epley manoeuvre can be undertaken if the symptoms return. If they have a lot of problems driving they should not do so until the condition has resolved.

REVISION PANEL

- The diagnosis of BPPV can typically be made on eliciting a classic history of vertigo lasting seconds occurring on head movement, with no other otological symptoms.
- BPPV diagnosis is confirmed by a positive Dix-Hallpike test.
- BPPV is treated by an Epley manoeuvre in the first instance.
- Classic BPPV is not associated with other intracranial pathology and the patient can be reassured of this.

ACUTE FACIAL PALSY

Questions

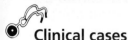 **Clinical cases**

For the clinical case scenario given

Q1: What is the likely differential diagnosis?
Q2: What additional features in the history would you like to elicit?
Q3: What is the important finding on examination?
Q4: What investigations would be most helpful and why?
Q5: What are the treatment options?

CASE 2.15 – **Acute facial palsy**

An adult aged 32 presents with a droopy face on the left side.

ＮＮ OSCE Counselling case

OSCE COUNSELLING CASE 2.14 – **A patient who has an acute Bell's palsy that is partial and occurred 3 days previously is concerned about recovery. What is your advice?**

Key concepts

- Assess upper and lower motor neuron function.
- House-Brackmann classification of facial nerve palsy
  I.   Normal
  II. Mild dysfunction
       - *Gross:*   Slight weakness on close inspection; may have synkinesis
       - *Motion:* Forehead – moderate to good, eye – complete closure with effort, mouth – slightly weak on maximal effort
  III. Moderate dysfunction
       - *Gross:*   Obvious, but not disfiguring between sides; noticeable but not severe synkinesis or spasm; at rest normal symmetry and tone
       - *Motion:* Forehead – slight to moderate movement, eye – complete closure with effort, mouth – slightly weak with maximal effort
  IV. Moderately severe
       - *Gross:*   Obvious weakness and/or disfiguring asymmetry; at rest normal symmetry and tone
       - *Motion:* Forehead – none, eye – incomplete closure, mouth – asymmetry with maximal effort
  V.   Severe dysfunction
       - *Gross:*   Only barely perceptible motion; at rest, asymmetry
       - *Motion:* Forehead – none, eye – incomplete closure, mouth – slight movement
  VI. Total paralysis
- No movement at all
- Corticosteroids demonstrated to improve the outcome from a facial palsy if begun within 2 weeks of onset
- Antivirals may be beneficial

Answers

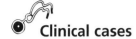
Clinical cases

CASE 2.15 – **Acute facial palsy**

A1: What is the likely differential diagnosis?
Bell's palsy is a diagnosis of exclusion.

A2: What additional features in the history would you like to elicit?
Ask whether the palsy came on suddenly and whether it is painful, particularly pain in the ear. Ask about hearing, taste and lacrimation.

A3: What is the important finding on examination?
Perform an otoneurological examination plus audiometry. Examine the neck for parotid masses.

Determine whether it is an upper or a lower motor neuron lesion – upper motor neuron lesions spare the forehead. The vast majority at this age will be lower motor neuron lesions. Try to grade the palsy. If you cannot determine the severity, note whether it is partial or complete.

Lower motor neuron facial nerve palsies can be caused by pathology in the following:

- Cerebellopontine (CP) angle – typically acoustic neuromas (see Case 2.10)
- Middle ear – temporal bone fracture, acute otitis media, cholesteatoma
- Parotid – malignant parotid neoplasms
- Globally – Bell's palsy, Ramsey Hunt, Lyme disease

Hence the diagnosis of Bell's palsy is a diagnosis of exclusion. Middle-ear conditions can be excluded by a combination of history and otoscopic findings. Parotid pathology can be excluded by neck palpation. The CP angle lesions cannot be excluded initially, and if there is no complete resolution of symptoms within 3 months then an MRI is undertaken. The presence of pain and vesicles on the soft palate, tonsil area, or ear canal and drum are diagnostic of Ramsay Hunt syndrome. This is the sensory supply of the seventh cranial nerve. Lyme disease may present with bilateral facial palsies with a history of exposure to the tick of *Borrelia* species. If all of the above is normal, then a presumptive diagnosis of Bell's is made.

The single most important observation is whether the patient can cover the cornea when she tries to close her eyes. The eye is most at risk from corneal damage with a facial palsy. Lacrimation may well be reduced as well.

A4: What investigations would be most helpful and why?
A simple case of Bell's palsy requires no investigation except audiometry. If the palsy does not improve completely after 3 months, then an MRI is required to exclude an acoustic neuroma.

A5: What are the treatment options?
Corticosteroids have been demonstrated to improve the outcome from a facial palsy if begun within 2 weeks of onset. Antivirals may be beneficial. The most important aspect of treatment is corneal protection. If there is any doubt, the patient should be referred to the eye surgeon. In the meantime artificial tears and tape, to ensure the eye remains closed at night, should be provided.

OSCE Counselling case

OSCE COUNSELLING CASE 2.14 – **A patient who has an acute Bell's palsy that is partial and occurred 3 days previously is concerned about recovery. What is your advice?**

Approximately 95 per cent of Bell's palsies recover completely by 9 months. If the palsy is partial and there is good eye closure, the recovery may well be quicker, often a few weeks. Some patients are concerned that they have had a stroke and you will be able to reassure them that this is not the case (a cerebrovascular accident (CVA) would present with an upper motor neuron lesion). Others may be concerned that there is something serious going on within the brain, and again you can stress that it is the nerve that supplies the face that is affected rather than anything more serious.

REVISION PANEL

- Evaluation of facial nerve palsies includes both determining the degree of the palsy and examining the course of the facial nerve to establish an underlying cause.
- Symptomatic treatment of the eye requires artificial tears and taping the eye closed at night.
- Bell's palsies resolve completely in 95 per cent of patients; this success rate is achieved if oral corticosteroids are administered within the first 2 weeks of onset.
- If the palsy does not resolve completely, an MRI of the course of the facial nerve is required.

THROAT

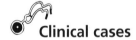

Questions

Clinical cases

For each of the clinical case scenarios given

Q1: What is the likely differential diagnosis?
Q2: What additional features in the history would you like to elicit?
Q3: What is the important finding on examination?
Q4: What investigations would be most helpful and why?
Q5: What are the treatment options?

CASE 2.16 – **Child with sore throat**

A mother presents with a child who has a recurrent sore throat causing constitutional symptoms.

CASE 2.17 – **Adolescent with acute sore throat**

An adolescent aged 17 comes to the surgery with an acute sore throat, feeling unwell.

CASE 2.18 – **Smoker with continuous sore throat**

A smoker aged 65 presents with a continuous sore throat, which is progressive, and complains of pain when swallowing.

OSCE Counselling case

OSCE COUNSELLING CASE 2.15 – **A mother wonders when a child may return to school after a tonsillectomy**

Key concepts

- Children have frequent viral respiratory infections.
- Tonsillitis causing persistent school absences for at least 1 year should be considered before a tonsillectomy is performed.
- Adolescents may have infectious mononucleosis.
- Smokers with sore throat and pain on swallowing may have a carcinoma.

Answers

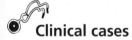 **Clinical cases**

CASE 2.16 – **Child with sore throat**

A1: What is the likely differential diagnosis?

Tonsillitis

A2: What additional features in the history would you like to elicit?

As children have frequent sore throat, it is important to determine whether the symptoms are the result of tonsillitis or simply a sore throat. This can be achieved by determining whether the tonsils swell up and have exudate on them during an attack. Establish the length and frequency of the attacks; they should last between 5 and 7 days and cause constitutional symptoms, and there should be six or more attacks a year resulting in school absence. The vast majority of other sore throats are caused by viral infections. Appetite may be affected intermittently and respiratory symptoms may also occur. Occasionally, there is obstructive sleep apnoea in patients with snoring. Sleep apnoea occurs mostly below 4 years of age.

A3: What is the important finding on examination?

Confirm tonsillitis with examination of the oral cavity. Cervical lymphadenopathy may be palpated and is frequent in children, particularly in the jugular digastric region.

A4: What investigations would be most helpful and why?

None is usually required.

A5: What are the treatment options?

As the vast majority of infections are viral, no treatment is required. Occasionally, bacterial tonsillitis does occur and if the symptoms are particularly severe and prolonged a 5-day course of antibiotics, such as amoxicillin, may be helpful. Tonsillectomy should not be recommended as the treatment unless the child has had seven episodes of tonsillitis in 1 year, or five episodes per year for 2 years, or three episodes per year for 3 years.

CASE 2.17 – **Adolescent with acute sore throat**

A1: What is the likely differential diagnosis?

Infectious mononucleosis (glandular fever) caused by Epstein-Barr virus

A2: What additional features in the history would you like to elicit?

A similar history should be taken to exclude recurrent tonsillitis. Concentrate on constitutional symptoms and contacts with a similar problem.

A3: What is the important finding on examination?

Examine the oral cavity and tonsil region and palpate the neck. Large fleshy tonsils with an exudate encroaching onto the soft palate may indicate infectious mononucleosis. Lymphadenopathy is often particularly severe and may extend from the neck to the rest of the body. Hepatosplenomegaly, pancreatitis and jaundice are rare complications of the condition.

A4: What investigations would be most helpful and why?

FBC which usually shows a monocytosis, and serology for glandular fever

A5: What are the treatment options?

The vast majority require little more than symptomatic treatment. Patients are advised to refrain from contact sports for 3 months after resolution of symptoms as there is an increased risk of hepatic or splenic injury if the liver or spleen is enlarged. Occasionally, patients with severe airway problems may require a course of oral steroids to reduce the lymphadenopathy but should be managed in hospital. Very occasionally an urgent tonsillectomy is required for airway management.

CASE 2.18 – **Smoker with continuous sore throat**

A1: What is the likely differential diagnosis?

Squamous cell carcinoma of the pharynx

A2: What additional features in the history would you like to elicit?

Particular attention should be paid to the progressive nature of the sore throat, oral intake and respiratory symptoms, including cough, sputum and haemoptysis. The history suggests a supraglottic carcinoma infiltrating the muscle that causes pain on swallowing.

A3: What is the important finding on examination?

Examine the oral cavity, neck and chest. If you can, undertake an endoscopic examination of the postnasal space, larynx and pharynx. The tonsil, supraglottic or laryngeal sites are the most likely. Ten per cent of smokers have more than one carcinoma in the aerodigestive tract. Oral examination may well not be conclusive. Examination of the neck will help stage the disease.

A4: What investigations would be most helpful and why?

These patients require screening investigations including an FBC, liver function tests, ECG and chest radiograph. Special investigation may include imaging of the neck and chest with CT and MRI. Biopsy the lesion and stage the tumour under general anaesthesia.

A5: What are the treatment options?

Depending on the tumour location and stage, radiotherapy or surgical resection and reconstruction are potential options.

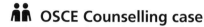 OSCE Counselling case

OSCE COUNSELLING CASE 2.15 – **A mother wonders when a child may return to school after a tonsillectomy**

Advise that it is usual for a child to stay off school for 2 weeks after surgery. Emphasize that the area has to heal and that there may be a secondary bleed as the slough comes away from the tonsillar fossa. Infection makes this worse, so children should be kept at home during the recovery period. Eating and drinking reduce the risk of infection as well.

REVISION PANEL

- Recurrent tonsillitis is a common presenting complaint. Assessment requires confirmation that tonsillitis is the underlying problem and determination of the number of episodes per year the child is suffering.
- Tonsillectomy can be a useful intervention if the underlying problem is recurrent tonsillitis and the above-mentioned frequency criteria are met.
- Glandular fever requires serology testing to confirm the diagnosis. It is typically a self-limiting condition; however, recovery takes longer than bacterial tonsillitis.
- A progressive dysphagia may well be the presenting complaint of a carcinoma. A full ENT examination should be performed, including staging imaging.

DIFFICULTY IN SWALLOWING

Questions

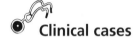
Clinical cases

For each of the clinical case scenarios given

> **Q1:** What is the likely differential diagnosis?
> **Q2:** What additional features in the history would you like to elicit?
> **Q3:** What should one look for in the examination?
> **Q4:** What investigations would be most helpful and why?
> **Q5:** What are the treatment options?

CASE 2.19 – **Lump in throat**

A woman aged 45 presents with an intermittent feeling of a lump in the throat.

CASE 2.20 – **Problems with swallowing**

A man aged 68 presents with continuous and progressive problems with swallowing. He is able to swallow liquids but finds solids more difficult.

░░ OSCE Counselling case

OSCE COUNSELLING CASE 2.16 – **What advice would you give to a patient with globus pharyngeus who is concerned that he might have a neoplasm?**

Key concepts

- Intermittent dysphagia with a constant weight is due to a benign condition.
- Continual dysphagia with weight loss may be malignant.
- Pain and discomfort are poorly localized in the embryological foregut and may present as a sensation of a neck lump.

Answers

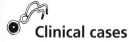
Clinical cases

CASE 2.19 – **Lump in throat**

CASE 2.20 – **Problems with swallowing**

A1: What is the likely differential diagnosis?

In both cases the differential diagnosis is either

- Globus pharyngeus – 'lump in one's throat' – that is the persistent sensation of having phlegm, a pill or some other sort of obstruction in the throat when there is none
- Neoplasm arising from either outside or within the oesophagus or pharynx (A pharyngeal pouch can cause dysphagia, although the hallmark is regurgitation of food.)

A2: What additional features in the history would you like to elicit?

Ask the same questions for both cases. Try to unravel whether there is a serious problem for the basis of the complaint. Ask whether there has been any weight change or any symptoms of reflux. Compression and direct erosion may come from the thyroid gland and rarely from the thoracic cavity contents and eventual ulceration. Smoking and alcohol consumption are risk factors for squamous cell carcinoma and their usage should be determined.

A3: What should one look for in the examination?

Palpate the neck – there is a physical sign called 'Toynbee's sign'. Move the laryngeal cartilages from side to side over the vertebral column. This produces crepitus in the normal individual and a post-cricoid carcinoma will lift the larynx forwards and crepitus is absent. This also occurs in foreign body or abscesses such as tuberculosis cold abscesses. Check for lymphadenopathy. In the ENT clinic, nasendoscopy with a flexible endoscope may show pooling of saliva or an abnormality such as a space-occupying lesion. In patients with globus there is no abnormality.

A4: What investigations would be most helpful and why?

These include an FBC (sideropenic dysphagia). If a patient is severely dehydrated with neoplasm, urea and electrolytes (U&Es) may be indicated. A barium swallow may show both reflux and neoplasia, but high lesions in the oesophagus do not show up well. Patients with globus should have fibreoptic gastro-oesophagoscopy. Perform a direct endoscopy and biopsy under general anaesthesia if in any doubt. Any tumour should be assessed, biopsied and staged.

A5: What are the treatment options?

The management depends on the nature of the underlying lesion and, for globus pharyngeus patients, simple reassurance is often enough. Reflux oesophagitis should be treated appropriately and is best managed in general practice. Neoplasms require a combination of excision, reconstruction and radiotherapy, or palliation.

⚭ OSCE Counselling case

OSCE COUNSELLING CASE 2.16 – **What advice would you give to a patient with globus pharyngeus who is concerned that he might have a neoplasm?**

Stress that intermittent problems are rarely serious and a stationary weight argues against a serious problem. Say also that the endoscopy has almost certainly excluded a neoplasm. A hiatus hernia and reflux may cause a sensation of a lump in the neck. The primitive foregut extends to the second part of the duodenum and takes its nerve supply with it – it is referred to the neck. Another feature of reflux is spasm of the cricopharyngeus sphincter. An explanation of these anatomical and functional reasons will result in acceptance of the condition and hopefully its cessation.

REVISION PANEL

- Diagnosing dysphagia and globus pharyngeus requires a constant vigilance to ensure the patient does not have a neoplasm.
- Patients who are smokers and drinkers are at increased risk of head and neck cancer.
- If the patient has intermittent symptoms, is a non-smoker, does not drink alcohol, has no loss of weight and examination is normal, globus pharyngeus is likely.
- Any patient who deviates from the above 'classic globus' patient may benefit from a direct laryngoscopy and upper oesophagoscopy to exclude a carcinoma.

HOARSE VOICE

Questions

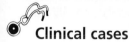

Clinical cases

For each of the clinical case scenarios given

> **Q1:** What is the likely differential diagnosis?
> **Q2:** What additional features in the history would you like to elicit?
> **Q3:** What is the important finding on examination?
> **Q4:** What investigations would be most helpful and why?
> **Q5:** What are the treatment options?

CASE 2.21 – **Hoarse voice 1**

A female teacher aged 45 has an intermittent hoarse voice and is concerned that this may affect her job.

CASE 2.22 – **Hoarse voice 2**

A 63-year-old heavy smoker presents with a progressive hoarse voice of 6 weeks' duration.

OSCE Counselling case

OSCE COUNSELLING CASE 2.17 – **A woman with an intermittent hoarse voice is worried about her career as a teacher and her voice problem. What advice would you give?**

Key concepts

- Intermittent hoarse voice is benign.
- Continual hoarse voice in a smoker is malignant.
- Speech and language therapy should be tried before surgery in benign conditions.
- Smokers may have more than one neoplasm.

Answers

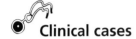

Clinical cases

CASE 2.21 – **Hoarse voice 1**

A1: What is the likely differential diagnosis?
Vocal cord nodules, muscle tension dysphonia and laryngopharyngeal reflux

A2: What additional features in the history would you like to elicit?
Ask about the nature of the job and when the hoarseness comes on. See whether the voice goes back to normal. If it is intermittent and comes on during the day, or during times of persistent voice use, it is almost certainly benign. Find out about hobbies such as singing. Ask about stress and the voice. Enquire about the symptoms of hiatus hernia and thyroid disease, and also whether the patient smokes or has chest disease such as asthma. Ask about nasal symptoms and snoring because this may dry the throat. Sinusitis is a rare cause of the problem and is often secondary to asthma and coughing.

A3: What is the important finding on examination?
Examination of the neck is usually uneventful. A flexible nasendoscopy in the clinic may show how the vocal apparatus is working and whether there are any lesions on the vocal cords. Singers' nodules are a sign of vocal misuse and occasionally a unilateral vocal cord polyp may be found. Bilateral diffuse oedema suggests chronic persistent abuse but may be found in conditions such as thyroid disease. In patients with laryngopharyngeal reflux the posterior larynx appears inflamed. Muscle tension dysphonia is a common problem in professional voice users and leads to insufficient adduction of the cords on phonation.

A4: What investigations would be most helpful and why?
These are rarely needed but do include an FBC and thyroid function tests.

A5: What are the treatment options?
Vocal hygiene should be practiced, such as frequent drinks to keep the larynx moist (not alcohol). Refrain from smoking if the patient is a smoker. Trials have shown that speech and language therapy is effective. Surgery is occasionally needed in patients with hoarseness. If the patient has asthma, therapy may improve the voice but sometimes the irritation is the result of the inhalers, or *Candida* species, on the vocal cords.

CASE 2.22 – **Hoarse voice 2**

A1: What is the likely differential diagnosis?

Carcinoma of nasopharynx/larynx

A2: What additional features in the history would you like to elicit?

The history should be taken similar to that in the previous case. The smoking history is most important here. Progressive hoarseness that lasts longer than 6 weeks is most likely to be a neoplasm. Examination of the neck is often uneventful because secondary nodes rarely occur in a simple carcinoma of the larynx as it presents relatively early.

A3: What is the important finding on examination?

Examination of the larynx will show a laryngeal cancer. This is classified by the TNM (tumours, node, metastases) classification, which helps to determine the treatment.

A4: What investigations would be most helpful and why?

A neck and chest CT should always be taken because secondary neoplasm in the chest occurs in 10 per cent of patients, this also aids in staging the disease. Similarly, an FBC, U&Es and liver function tests, together with thyroid function tests, may be required before radiotherapy or surgery.

A5: What are the treatment options?

Treatment depends on the TNM classification. Very small malignant squamous cell tumours can be removed with LASER once a biopsy has confirmed it. These patients should be followed up closely. The conventional treatment for small tumours is radiotherapy. However, this results in disability to the larynx and pharynx, with dryness and soreness as well as mucositis, and is best given in a fractionated regimen over a 6-week period rather than a shorter one. Larger tumours require surgery and radiotherapy. There is a move at present to more conservative surgery rather than laryngectomy and block dissection.

OSCE Counselling case

OSCE COUNSELLING CASE 2.17 – **A woman with an intermittent hoarse voice is worried about her career as a teacher and her voice problem. What advice would you give?**

Explain that voice care and rest are the most appropriate treatment. Whispering strains the voice more than talking normally. Avoid singing and shouting. Stress the value of speech and language therapy, which allows voice training and counselling at the same time. The voice may return to normal.

REVISION PANEL

- Intermittent hoarseness, especially in non-smokers, is typically benign and can be confirmed endoscopically.
- Benign hoarseness responds well to speech therapy and improved vocal hygiene.
- Progressive hoarseness, especially in smokers, is likely to represent malignant disease.
- Malignant neoplasms of the larynx are managed by confirmation of diagnosis (by biopsy) followed by staging of the disease (by clinic examination and imaging).

PAINLESS NECK LUMP

Questions

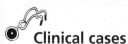

Clinical cases

For each of the clinical case scenarios given

Q1: What is the likely differential diagnosis?
Q2: What additional features in the history would you like to elicit?
Q3: What should one look for in the examination?
Q4: What investigations would be most helpful and why?
Q5: What are the treatment options?

CASE 2.23 – **Painless neck lump 1**

A woman aged 52 has just returned from India and has noticed a painless lump in the mid cervical region.

CASE 2.24 – **Painless neck lump 2**

A Chinese man aged 33 presents with a painless left jugulodigastric swelling.

⁙ OSCE Counselling case

OSCE COUNSELLING CASE 2.18 – **The woman who has had the neck biopsy that shows TB returns to clinic. What advice would you give her?**

Key concepts

- Lymph nodes >2 cm are abnormal.
- Painless neck lumps in Asians are frequently tuberculosis (TB).
- Painless neck lumps in Chinese adults are often postnasal space squamous cell carcinoma metastases.
- Always undertake a fine-needle aspiration sample for cytology before surgery.
- Lymphoma and carcinoma may occur.
- Reactive lymph node swelling is the most common cause.

Answers

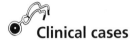
Clinical cases

CASE 2.23 – **Painless neck lump 1**

A1: What is the likely differential diagnosis?

Tuberculosis, laryngeal/pharyngeal carcinoma

A2: What additional features in the history would you like to elicit?

Determine whether there are any night sweats, rigors or any other features of TB such as respiratory symptoms. Ask direct questions about difficulty in swallowing, voice changes or any other constitutional symptoms – indicating laryngeal/pharyngeal carcinoma. Enquire about any family history/social contacts with TB.

A3: What should one look for in the examination?

Examination of the neck will often reveal that there is a collection of nodes that are discrete and rubbery, but not attached to the skin or deeper structures. Measure the size because a node >2 cm diameter is always trouble. A lymphoma may feel the same. A full ENT examination including visualization of the larynx and pharynx should also be undertaken.

A4: What investigations would be most helpful and why?

FBC, Mantoux test, chest radiograph and fine-needle aspiration (FNA) of the neck lump are useful. Undertake excision biopsy with histology and culture after the result of the FNA cytology.

A5: What are the treatment options?

The treatment depends on the nature of the lesion. The most likely cause of this type of lesion is a tuberculous node. The key point in management is to undertake an FNA before one goes to excision biopsy as FNA can direct the appropriate treatment early on. If TB is suspected an open biopsy with both culture and histology is required. Acid-fast bacilli may be exceptionally difficult to identify on histological specimens and grown only on culture. However, if the diagnosis is suspected, it is important to notify the authorities and to send the patient for appropriate antituberculous chemotherapy.

CASE 2.24 – **Painless neck lump 2**

A1: What is the likely differential diagnosis?

Postnasal space squamous cell carcinoma

A2: What additional features in the history would you like to elicit?

Ask which part of China the patient is from because patients from southern China have a high risk of postnasal space carcinoma. Ask about nasal symptoms such as nose bleeding and blockage of the nose. Ask about neurological symptoms such as numbness of the face. Undertake a general history.

A3: What should one look for in the examination?

Perform a full head and neck examination including full nasendoscopy. It is important to visualize the postnasal space in all patients with upper cervical lesions that might be neoplastic. The cranial nerves should be examined carefully; numbness of the cheek is particularly important, as is any degree of proptosis.

A4: What investigations would be most helpful and why?

Full blood count, U&Es, liver function tests, CT of the postnasal space and FNA cytology of the neck lump

A5: What are the treatment options?

If the diagnosis is a postnasal space carcinoma, treatment is by radiotherapy plus a neck dissection together with radiotherapy to the neck fields. A third of patients present with nasal symptoms, a third with cervical metastases and a third with intracranial extension. This tumour can be particularly aggressive. It occurs in a younger age group and is associated with the Epstein Barr virus (EBV). Levels of the immunoglobulin IgA to EBV may indicate recurrent disease.

♟♞ OSCE Counselling case

OSCE COUNSELLING CASE 2.18 – **The woman who has had the neck biopsy that shows TB returns to clinic. What advice would you give her?**

Explain that TB is eminently treatable and that the chest physician or infectious diseases doctor will be treating her. Say also that it will be important to screen the family to make sure that no other family members have the disease and that if they do they will have to be treated. This should eradicate the condition and the patient should be well for many years.

REVISION PANEL

- The most common cause of cervical lymphadenopathy is reactive, this is typically related to an underlying infection (acne, tonsillitis).
- Painless lymphadenopathy especially if >2 cm is always concerning.
- History and examination should focus at determining the underlying cause and excluding laryngeal and pharyngeal carcinoma.
- A FNA of cervical lymphadenopathy should always be performed.
- Cross-sectional imaging can aid in determining the extent of disease and assist with diagnosis.

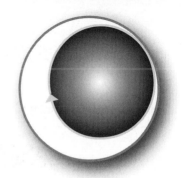

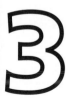

3 Ophthalmology

Desirée Murray

OPHTHALMOLOGY

OPHTHALMOLOGY

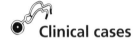

Clinical cases

For each of the clinical case scenarios given

Q1: What is the differential diagnosis?
Q2: What issues in the history support the diagnosis?
Q3: What additional features in the history would you seek to support a particular
diagnosis?
Q4: What clinical examination would you perform and why?
Q5: What investigations would be most helpful and why?
Q6: What treatment options are appropriate?

CASE 3.1 – 'I have pain in my eye and I can't see with it'

A 65-year-old woman presents with a 1-day history of pain, redness and reduced vision in one eye. She
has worn spectacles for reading since the age of 7 years.

CASE 3.2 – 'I have suddenly lost the vision in one eye, but I have no pain'

A 50-year-old patient presents with a 1-day history of sudden painless loss of vision. The patient has
diabetes and hypertension.

CASE 3.3 – 'I have flashing lights and floaters in one eye'

A 40-year-old patient gives a 1-week history of sudden-onset flashing lights and floaters in one eye. The
patient has worn distance spectacles since the age of 12 years.

CASE 3.4 – 'My vision has gradually become cloudy and dim, but there is no pain in my eye'

A 60-year-old patient complains of a gradual deterioration in vision in both eyes over 1 year.

CASE 3.5 – 'I have difficulty seeing at night'

A 35-year-old patient presents with a 1-year history of difficulty seeing at night. The patient also
complains of constriction of the visual field.

CASE 3.6 – 'I have double vision'

A 60-year-old patient presents with a 1-week history of double vision.

CASE 3.7 – 'I have intermittent loss of vision in one eye for a few seconds and then my vision returns'

A 50-year-old patient complains of intermittent loss of vision in one eye like a 'cloud' or 'curtain' descending over the vision, which clears after a few seconds.

CASE 3.8 – 'I have intermittent loss of vision in both eyes and then my vision clears'

A 30-year-old woman complains of episodes of visual loss in both eyes associated with eye movements. She has a 1-month history of intermittent headache.

CASE 3.9 – 'My child's eye has a turn'

A parent complains that her 2-year-old infant has developed a turn in one eye.

CASE 3.10 – 'My baby has watery eyes'

A mother complains that her 4-month-old baby has had watery eyes since birth.

ii OSCE Counselling cases

OSCE COUNSELLING CASE 3.1 – 'Why am I having difficulty reading since having my cataract surgery?'

A 60-year-old patient recently had uncomplicated cataract extraction with an intraocular lens implant. The patient complains of difficulty reading. The distance vision is good. The patient has not yet obtained new spectacles.

> Can you reassure the patient? Explain why the patient is experiencing problems with unaided near vision and what can be done to correct the problem.

OSCE COUNSELLING CASE 3.2 – 'Why can't I see as well now as I did after my cataract surgery 18 months ago?'

A 60-year-old patient had successful cataract surgery 18 months ago. The patient complains of gradual reduction in vision in the pseudophakic eye. There is no history of diabetes or hypertension. Ocular examination is normal apart from the presence of posterior capsule opacification.

> What is posterior capsule opacification? Explain this condition to the patient, including its treatment.

OSCE COUNSELLING CASE 3.3 – 'Why am I short of breath since starting treatment for glaucoma?'

This 60-year-old-patient has been diagnosed with glaucoma. He was prescribed timolol 0.5 per cent eyedrops.

> Is it possible to develop dyspnoea in association with timolol use? Discuss the possible side effects of this eyedrop.

OSCE COUNSELLING CASE 3.4 – 'I have recently been diagnosed with glaucoma. Can I still drive?'

> Adequate standards of vision must be met for all drivers. Suitability to drive should be considered at every consultation. Driving may be continued as long as the patient has been confirmed to meet the visual acuity standard and recommended national guidelines for visual field. Any advice given should be well documented in the patient's medical record.

OSCE COUNSELLING CASE 3.5 – 'I have well-controlled diabetes. I have no problems with my vision. I had my eyes checked 1 year ago. When should I next have my eyes examined?'

This 50-year-old patient has had diabetes for 5 years. The patient has normal distance (6/6) and reading (N5) vision with glasses.

> Explain to the patient why he needs a complete eye examination, including dilated funduscopy to screen for diabetic retinopathy, at least once a year, in spite of normal vision. What factors would you consider important when counselling this patient?

OSCE COUNSELLING CASE 3.6 – 'Will laser treatment make my vision worse? My neighbour, who also has diabetes, is now blind following laser treatment'

This patient has had type 2 diabetes for 10 years. The ophthalmologist has recommended laser treatment for her right eye.

What factors would you consider important when counselling this patient?

Glossary of terms

Age-related macular degeneration (ARMD)	• Non-exudative ARMD – dry type: age-related macular changes characterized by discrete whitish-yellow spots identified as drusen, pigment changes (hyperpigmentration and hypopigmentation) and atrophy of the retinal pigment epithelium.
	• Exudative ARMD – wet type: manifestations of choroidal neovascularization and/or accumulation of fluid or blood beneath the retinal pigment epithelium in a patient with age-related maculopathy.
Amblyopia	Decreased visual acuity without detectable organic disease of the eye or visual pathway, the eye having not developed normal vision during early childhood..
Anisocoria	Condition in which the pupils of the two eyes are of different sizes.
Astigmatism	An optical condition in which the refractive power of the eye varies in different meridians, usually caused by the cornea having a greater curvature in one direction than in another (similar to a rugby ball as opposed to the more even shape of a football). As a result, parallel rays of light do not focus at a point and a distinct retinal image cannot form. It may be associated with long-sightedness, short-sightedness or both.
Cryotherapy	Procedure carried out with a freezing probe.
Cycloplegic refraction	Paralysis of the ciliary muscle by means of drugs, thus allowing measurement of the refractive error uncomplicated by changes in accommodation.
Dacryocystitis	Inflammation of the lacrimal sac.
Dacryocystorhinostomy	Surgical procedure to (re-)establish lacrimal drainage.
Dacryostenosis	Atresia of the nasolacrimal duct.
Degenerative (pathological) myopia	Abnormality in which the axial length of the eye is excessive. There is patchy choroidal atrophy. The sclera is bared in the region surrounding the optic nerve and at the macula, and the choroid is easily visible.
Electroretinogram	Action potential that follows stimulation of the retina.
Enophthalmos	Recession of the eye within the orbit.
Exophthalmos	Abnormal protrusion of one or both eyes. The term is often used when there is an association with thyroid dysfunction.
Fundus fluorescein angiography	Intravenous sodium fluorescein combined with serial black and white photography to study the retinal circulation.
Hypermetropia/hyperopia/ long-sightedness/ far-sightedness	Condition in which parallel rays of light are brought to a point focus behind the retina, because the eye is too short for its own focusing power.
Hypopyon	Pus in the anterior chamber.
Iridotomy	Opening through all layers of the iris.

Iritis	Inflammation of the iris.
Keratitis	Inflammation of the cornea.
Leukocoria	White pupillary reflex.
Myopia/short-sightedness/ near-sightedness	Condition in which parallel rays of light are brought to a point focus in front of the retina, because the eye is too long for its own focusing power.
Nasolacrimal duct	Duct that connects the lower end of the lacrimal sac with the inferior meatus of the nose.
Posterior synechiae	Adhesions between the iris and the lens.
Posterior vitreous detachment	Separation of the peripheral vitreous from the retina.
Presbyopia	Loss of accommodation as a result of loss of elasticity of the lens with increasing age, so that the near point recedes. The inability to focus for near results in most people aged over 40 years needing reading spectacles.
Proptosis	Protrusion of the eyeball.
Relative afferent pupillary defect	Transmission defect of the optic nerve demonstrated by the 'swinging flashlight test'. When light is directed into the eye on the normal side both pupils react to light. When light is quickly switched to the abnormal side, the pupil, instead of remaining constricted (from the consensual reaction), dilates despite the light stimulation.
Rods	Light-sensitive elements of the retina that function at low levels of illumination. They are the main photoreceptors of the peripheral retina.
Scintillations	Visual hallucinations with flashing lights occurring in occipital lobe disorders, particularly migraine.
Scleritis	Inflammation of the sclera.
Trabeculectomy	A filtering operation for glaucoma, by creation of a fistula between the anterior chamber of the eye and the subconjunctival space.
Uveitis	Inflammation of the uveal tract.

Answers

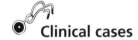 **Clinical cases**

CASE 3.1 – 'I have pain in my eye and I can't see with it'

A1: What is the differential diagnosis?

- Acute angle-closure glaucoma
- Iritis (anterior uveitis)
- Keratitis – bacterial, viral, autoimmune peripheral ulcerative keratitis (PUK)
- Scleritis/sclerokeratitis

A2: What issues in the history support the diagnosis?

The history of having worn reading spectacles since childhood suggests long-sightedness (hyperopia) (Figure 3.1). This increases the risk of developing acute angle-closure glaucoma because patients who are long-sighted have small eyes with crowded anterior segments and narrow drainage angles.

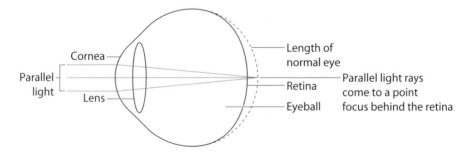

Figure 3.1 Hypermetropia or hyperopia: long-sightedness.

A3: What additional features in the history would you seek to support a particular diagnosis?

It is important to enquire about symptoms of haloes around lights and intermittent blurring of vision, which suggest previous episodes of increased intraocular pressure with corneal oedema. Previous attacks of angle closure may have resolved spontaneously. Is there any associated nausea and vomiting, as this is often the case in acute glaucoma?

Enquire about photophobia – often quite marked in patients with iritis. Is there a history of rheumatoid arthritis or other autoimmune disorder, which may be associated with PUK or scleritis?

Does the patient wear contact lenses? This may predispose to bacterial keratitis/corneal ulcer. Is there a history of herpetic disease (cold sores or previous herpes simplex keratitis)?

A4: What clinical examination would you perform and why?

Visual acuity should be measured. Examine the red reflex. A reduced or absent red reflex is found in corneal oedema. Compare the clarity of the cornea in the affected eye with that in the contralateral eye. Palpate the globe to determine whether the intraocular pressure is elevated, but be gentle because the eye may be quite tender. Examine the cornea with the aid of fluorescein dye and cobalt blue light, looking for staining, which would indicate corneal epithelial erosions, abrasion or ulcer. In patients with herpes simplex keratitis, the corneal ulcer assumes a typical branching pattern known as a dendritic ulcer. Pay attention to the distribution of the redness – circumcorneal injection is typical of iritis (ciliary flush), whereas with scleritis the eye may be diffusely injected or the redness may be localized to one segment of the sclera. Scleral nodules may also be present. Examine the pupil. A constricted pupil may indicate iritis whereas a fixed, mid-dilated, irregular pupil is seen in acute glaucoma. In severe iritis or bacterial keratitis, a hypopyon may be visible in the anterior chamber.

A5: What investigations would be most helpful and why?

It is important to examine the contralateral eye to determine whether the drainage angle is narrow. An elevated erythrocyte sedimentation rate (ESR) or packed cell volume (PCV) may indicate an underlying autoimmune or other systemic condition. Do a full blood count (FBC) to check for raised white cell count (WCC) (neutrophilia, lymphocytosis or monocytosis). Also do blood glucose to exclude diabetes, because this may sometimes be associated with iritis. A chest radiograph may detect signs of sarcoidosis or tuberculosis (TB).

A6: What treatment options are appropriate?

If the patient has acute glaucoma, treatment consists of the following:

- Medical treatment: antiglaucoma medications including pilocarpine 4 per cent and intravenous acetazolamide are administered. Pilocarpine eyedrops are instilled into the contralateral eye to minimize the risk of that eye developing acute angle-closure glaucoma.
- Laser treatment: Nd:YAG (neodymium:yttrium–aluminium–garnet) laser peripheral iridotomy (Figure 3.2) is performed when the corneal oedema clears sufficiently. Prophylactic YAG laser peripheral iridotomy is performed in the contralateral eye.
- If there is extensive damage to the anterior chamber drainage angle, ciliary body ablation with the diode laser is sometimes required to achieve a substantial reduction in intraocular pressure.
- Surgical treatment: sometimes glaucoma filtration surgery (trabeculectomy) (Figure 3.3) is necessary to control intraocular pressure.

If the patient has iritis, scleritis or infective keratitis, treatment consists of the following:

- Iritis is treated with topical steroid eyedrops.
- Scleritis is treated with oral non-steroidal anti-inflammatory drugs (NSAIDs), topical and/or systemic steroids or steroid-sparing immunosuppressive agents, as indicated.
- Autoimmune PUK is treated with systemic immunosuppression.
- Patients with intraocular inflammation should also be treated with cycloplegic eyedrops to dilate the pupil to prevent the development of posterior synechiae, and relax the ciliary muscle and reduce ocular discomfort and photophobia.
- Infective keratitis is treated with the appropriate anti-infective agent — antibacterial, antifungal, antiprotozoal, or antiviral. Bacterial corneal ulcers are treated with intensive topical antibiotics (after corneal scraping for culture and sensitivity). The dendritic ulcer of herpes simplex keratitis is treated with topical antiherpetics such as aciclovir or ganciclovir eye ointment.

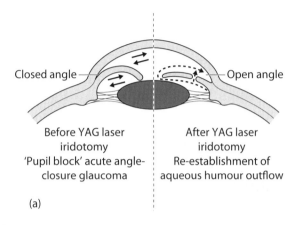

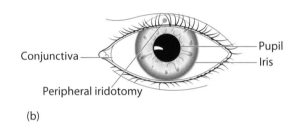

Figure 3.2 (a) Acute angle-closure glaucoma treated by Nd:YAG (neodymium:yttrium–aluminium–garnet) laser iridotomy. (b) Peripheral laser iridotomy.

CASE 3.2 – 'I have suddenly lost the vision in one eye, but I have no pain'

A1: What is the differential diagnosis?

- Central retinal artery occlusion
- Branch retinal artery occlusion
- Central retinal vein occlusion
- Branch retinal vein occlusion
- Ischaemic optic neuropathy
- Vitreous haemorrhage
- Retinal detachment
- ARMD (wet type)

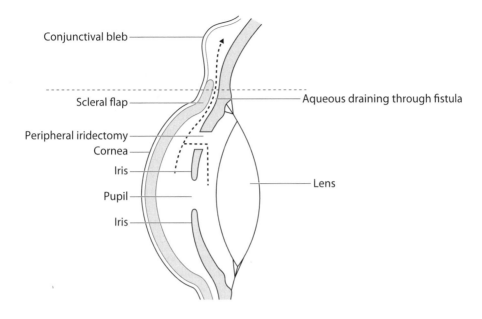

Conjunctival bleb

Scleral flap

Aqueous draining through fistula

Peripheral iridectomy
Cornea
Iris

Pupil

Iris

Lens

Figure 3.3 Trabeculectomy – glaucoma filtration surgery.

A2: What issues in the history support the diagnosis?

The fact that the patient has diabetes and hypertension should alert one to the possibility of diabetic retinopathy, other retinal vascular disease and/or carotid artery disease with embolic sequelae.

A3: What additional features in the history would you seek to support a particular diagnosis?

Ask about previous episodes of transient loss of vision, or transient ischaemic attacks (TIAs). Has the patient ever suffered a stroke or heart attack? Has the patient had retinal laser treatment in the past for diabetic retinopathy or macular degeneration? If the patient is short-sighted (myopic) (Figure 3.4) or there is a history of ocular trauma, the risk of retinal detachment is increased. Enquire about headache, scalp tenderness, proximal myalgia, jaw claudication, anorexia and weight loss – symptoms of giant cell arteritis. The drug history is important. Is the patient on any antiarrhythmic or anticoagulant medication for atrial fibrillation? Does the patient smoke?

A4: What clinical examination would you perform and why?

Measure the visual acuity. Examine the pupils for a relative afferent pupillary defect (RAPD). Examine the red reflex, which is reduced or absent in vitreous haemorrhage. Perform ophthalmoscopy. Look for evidence of diabetic retinopathy (retinal haemorrhages, hard exudates and cotton-wool spots), retinal vein occlusion (retinal haemorrhages and cotton-wool spots), retinal artery emboli (yellow refractile plaques at the bifurcation of retinal arterioles), 'cherry red spot' at the macula, optic disc swelling and superficial disc haemorrhages or retinal detachment. Macular haemorrhages and hard exudates may also be seen in 'wet' macular degeneration. Examine the cardiovascular system – pulse, blood pressure, cardiac murmur and carotid bruit.

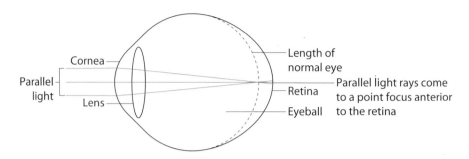

Figure 3.4 Myopia: short-sightedness.

A5: What investigations would be most helpful and why?

In the case of ischaemic optic neuropathy or retinal artery occlusion, an ESR, plasma viscosity (PV) and/or C-reactive protein (CRP) should be done to exclude giant cell arteritis. The blood sugar and the lipid profile need to be measured. Do an FBC to check for thrombocytopenia. Carotid Doppler ultrasonography should also be requested to determine the extent of carotid artery stenosis. Electrocardiography and echocardiography may be indicated.

A6: What treatment options are appropriate?

Treatment is aimed at improving visual prognosis in the affected eye, preventing a similar occurrence in the contralateral eye and reducing the risk of a major cardiovascular event.

- Medical treatment: giant cell arteritis is a medical emergency and the patient must be admitted for treatment with high-dose systemic steroids. Temporal artery biopsy may confirm the diagnosis. Retinal artery occlusions presenting within 4 to 6 hours of the onset of symptoms are ophthalmic emergencies, as this is generally accepted as the therapeutic time window. Urgent referral to the ophthalmology department is needed so that measures can be instituted to attempt to dislodge any retinal artery emboli. Blood pressure, blood sugar and serum lipids need to be controlled if elevated.
- Laser treatment: sometimes laser treatment is indicated for retinal neovascularization secondary to proliferative diabetic retinopathy or ischaemia after retinal vein or artery occlusion. Laser treatment is also indicated for macular oedema after retinal vein occlusion and for some cases of wet ARMD.
- Surgical treatment: temporal artery biopsy may be useful in confirming a diagnosis of giant cell arteritis. The patient should be referred to a vascular surgeon to determine whether carotid endarterectomy is indicated. The patient with a retinal detachment is referred to the ophthalmologist for surgical repair. Intravitreal injection of the antivascular endothelial growth factor (VEGF) agent Ranibizumab (Lucentis) is recommended as a treatment for wet age-related macular degeneration (AMD) in restricted circumstances (NICE Technology Appraisal 155). Bevacizumab (Avastin) is used off-label to treat eye conditions for which there are no licensed treatments, or in a minority of wet AMD cases where improvements in vision have not been achieved with Ranibizumab.

CASE 3.3 – 'I have flashing lights and floaters in one eye'

A1: What is the differential diagnosis?

- Posterior vitreous detachment (PVD)
- Retinal detachment (RD)
- Migraine

A2: What issues in the history support the diagnosis?

This history of having worn distance spectacles since childhood is evidence of short-sightedness (myopia) (Figure 3.4). Myopic patients are prone to PVD at a younger age than patients who are not myopic. They also have an increased risk of developing RD. Fortunately, most patients with a PVD do not develop RD, but the latter can be excluded only by detailed examination of the retina through a dilated pupil. A history of migraine may suggest that diagnosis for the present episode.

A3: What additional features in the history would you seek to support a particular diagnosis?

Ask about any noticeable visual field defect, often described by the patient as a shadow or dark patch in the peripheral vision. The triad of flashes, floaters and a field defect is very suspicious of RD. A history of ocular trauma increases its risk. Enquire about associated headache, nausea and vomiting suggestive of migraine. Scintillations lasting 15 to 20 minutes are virtually diagnostic of migraine.

A4: What clinical examination would you perform and why?

Visual acuity should be measured, and pupils assessed for RAPD. Dilated funduscopy is performed at the slit-lamp with a contact lens or by using the binocular indirect ophthalmoscope and indentation to visualize the peripheral retina.

A5: What investigations would be most helpful and why?

Examination of the contralateral eye to exclude asymptomatic retinal breaks or RD is important.

A6: What treatment options are appropriate?

- Reassurance: PVD in the absence of retinal breaks or RD does not require treatment.
- Medical treatment: migraine usually responds to appropriate analgesics.
- Laser treatment: retinal holes, tears or breaks may be treatable with laser if detected at an early stage.
- Surgical treatment: RD is referred to the ophthalmologist for surgical repair.

REVISION PANEL

- Nausea and vomiting in the presence of a painful red eye may be symptoms of primary (acute) angle-closure glaucoma
- Photophobia and circumcorneal injection may be indications of acute anterior uveitis (iritis).
- Contact lens wear predisposes to bacterial keratitis/corneal ulcers.
- Assessment of the pupils is important in the differential diagnosis of a painful red eye. In primary angle-closure glaucoma, the pupil is fixed and mid-dilated, whereas in acute iritis the pupil may be constricted.
- Fluorescein dye and the cobalt blue filter are essential components of a comprehensive anterior segment eye examination.
- Although underlying arteriosclerosis (diabetes, hypertension, hyperlipidaemia) is the main cause of retinal artery occlusion and ischaemic optic neuropathy, it is important to exclude vasculitis (for example, giant cell arteritis) in patients with sudden painless loss of vision.
- Relative afferent pupillary defect (RAPD) is an important sign of retinal or optic nerve pathology.
- Intravitreal injections of anti-VEGF agents are often used in the treatment of neovascular ocular conditions such as wet ARMD, central retinal vein occlusion and proliferative diabetic retinopathy. It is also used in the treatment of macular oedema secondary to retinal vein occlusions or diabetic maculopathy.
- The symptoms of posterior vitreous detachment and retinal detachment are identical. All patients with sudden onset flashes and floaters, especially in the presence of a peripheral visual field defect need to be referred for a detailed dilated fundus examination.
- Migraine may cause flashing lights and visual disturbance.

CASE 3.4 – 'My vision has gradually become cloudy and dim, but there is no pain in my eye'

A1: What is the differential diagnosis?

- Cataracts
- Age-related macular degeneration (dry type)
- Diabetic retinopathy
- Primary open-angle glaucoma.

A2: What issues in the history support the diagnosis?

The gradual and progressive onset of the visual loss is typical of cataract and dry ARMD.

A3: What additional features in the history would you seek to support a particular diagnosis?

Is the deterioration in vision for distance, near or both? Cataracts affect both, whereas ARMD and diabetic maculopathy may affect near vision to a greater extent than distance vision. Ask about a history of diabetes and hypertension. Does the patient smoke? Is there a family history of glaucoma?

A4: What clinical examination would you perform and why?

Measure the visual acuity. Examine the red reflex – this is reduced if there is nuclear sclerotic cataract. Intraocular pressure is measured. Ophthalmoscopy is performed looking for signs of ARMD and diabetic retinopathy, including retinal haemorrhages and hard exudates at the macula. Examine the optic disc closely. Note the disc colour, the contour of the disc margins and the cup:disc ratio. The cup:disc ratio is enlarged in primary open-angle glaucoma.

A5: What investigations would be most helpful and why?

If diabetic maculopathy is detected, the patient may require fundus fluorescein angiography. Fluorescein angiography may also be helpful in excluding wet ARMD, which may coexist with the dry type. The blood pressure, blood sugar and lipid profile are measured. Visual field analysis is performed if glaucoma is suspected.

A6: What treatment options are appropriate?

Unfortunately, there is no effective treatment for dry ARMD. Although prophylactic laser treatment has been tried, there is little evidence that this is of benefit. The Age-Related Eye Disease Study (AREDS) evaluated the effect of high doses of zinc and selected antioxidants (beta-carotene and vitamins C and E) and found significant reduction in the risk of progression in patients with advanced ARMD (categories 3 and 4). The results of the Age-Related Eye Disease Study 2 (AREDS2) show that taking the omega-3 fatty acids DHA and EPA as supplements did not reduce the risk of progression to advanced AMD. There may be benefits to substituting lutein/zeaxanthin for β-carotene in the original AREDS formulation, especially for current or former smokers, and for people who do not eat enough green leafy vegetables. However, because these benefits are based on subgroup analysis, they should be interpreted with caution.

Specific nutritional supplements are therefore indicated in advanced ARMD. The patient should also be advised to stop smoking. Arrangements for the provision of low visual aids (large-print material, optical aids and non-optical aids) and rehabilitation should be remembered.

- Medical treatment: in most cases, primary open-angle glaucoma is successfully treated with antiglaucoma eyedrops.
- Laser treatment: laser trabeculoplasty is sometimes used in the treatment of glaucoma. Laser treatment is performed for diabetic maculopathy, if there is clinically significant macular oedema.
- Surgical treatment: glaucoma filtration surgery (trabeculectomy) (Figure 3.3) or a glaucoma drainage device may become necessary if medical treatment is ineffective or not well tolerated. Visually significant cataract is treated by phacoemulsification and intraocular lens implant.

CASE 3.5 – 'I have difficulty seeing at night'

A1: What is the differential diagnosis?

- Retinitis pigmentosa (RP)
- Vitamin A deficiency
- Primary open-angle glaucoma
- Cataracts
- Degenerative myopia.
- Previous panretinal laser photocoagulation

A2: What issues in the history support the diagnosis?

Night blindness (nyctalopia) is a feature of many diseases. Vitamin A is necessary for the conversion of light energy to an electrical signal in the rod outer segments. The rods function at low levels of illumination, so vitamin A deficiency results in night blindness. Difficulty with night vision may indicate an abnormality of rod function and is characteristic of RP. However, any cause of extensive peripheral retinal degeneration, including primary open-angle glaucoma and degenerative myopia, results in peripheral visual field loss and poor night vision. Cataracts cause a general reduction in the amount of light entering the eye and can therefore produce similar symptoms.

A3: What additional features in the history would you seek to support a particular diagnosis?

It is important to determine the onset of symptoms. Patients with RP often begin having difficulty with night vision in the teenage years (e.g. they may report having had difficulty finding their way around a cinema or other dark environment). Does the patient have a hearing deficit? Usher's syndrome is a variation of RP that also impairs hearing. Ask about symptoms that may suggest constriction of the peripheral visual field, such as involvement in road traffic accidents. Is the patient myopic (short-sighted) (Figure 3.4)? Does the patient wear spectacles or contact lenses? The incidence of myopia is increased in RP. Ask about a family history of RP, night blindness, glaucoma and cataracts. Enquire about any history of abdominal surgery involving small bowel resection or liver disease, which may cause malabsorption and hypovitaminosis (vitamin A deficiency).

A4: What clinical examination would you perform and why?

Measure visual acuity and assess visual fields to confrontation. Examine the red reflex, which may be reduced in eyes with cataract. Posterior subcapsular cataract often occurs in patients with RP. Check the intraocular pressure. Dilated funduscopy may show the classic appearance of RP with pigment proliferation and accumulation of pigment shaped as bone corpuscles ('bone spicules') in the midperipheral retina. There may be diffuse large areas of chorioretinal atrophy in degenerative myopia. Examine the optic disc carefully for optic atrophy and/or pathological optic disc cupping (enlarged cup:disc ratio). Look for retinal arteriolar attenuation and cystoid macular oedema seen as a dull or absent foveal light reflex, because this may occur in patients with RP.

A5: What investigations would be most helpful and why?

In patients with RP or advanced glaucoma, visual field testing shows marked constriction of the peripheral field (tunnel vision). In RP, the electroretinogram is the most useful electrodiagnostic test. It is reduced in amplitude or non-recordable and helps to confirm the diagnosis. Cataracts are uncommon at such a young age and, if present, fasting blood sugar should be requested to exclude diabetes.

A6: What treatment options are appropriate?

In patients with RP, the eyes should be examined annually to determine the progression of the disease and to monitor for the development of cataract and glaucoma. Genetic counselling is mandatory. A complete family history and ophthalmological assessment of all family members will help to classify the disease as X-chromosome linked, autosomal dominant or autosomal recessive. Many patients with RP are legally blind in middle age and appropriate counselling must be given in collaboration with a geneticist.

- Counselling: unfortunately there is no treatment for degenerative myopia. Appropriate advice and support need to be organized.
- Medical treatment: there have been many different treatments suggested for RP, ranging from vitamin A in high doses to retinal electrostimulation, but to date none has been effective. Small doses of vitamins A and E may be appropriate but the recommended daily allowance should not be exceeded.
- Primary open-angle glaucoma is treated medically with antiglaucoma eyedrops.
- Laser treatment: argon or selective laser trabeculoplasty is sometimes useful in controlling intraocular pressure in patients with glaucoma.
- Surgical treatment: glaucoma filtration surgery (trabeculectomy) (Figure 3.3) may be necessary to lower intraocular pressure effectively.
- Visually significant cataract is treated by phacoemulsification cataract extraction and intraocular lens implant.

REVISION PANEL

- Gradual progressive painless loss of vision is a common complaint among the aging population. Although cataract is a common diagnosis, it is important to exclude coexisting conditions such as age-related macular degeneration, diabetic retinopathy and glaucoma.
- The Age-Related Eye Disease studies (AREDS and AREDS2) have provided evidence that dietary supplements reduce the risk of progression of advanced (categories 3 and 4) dry ARMD.
- Liver disease or abdominal surgery involving small bowel resection may cause malabsorption and hypovitaminosis, including vitamin A deficiency, which could result in difficulty with night vision.
- Night blindness may be caused by any peripheral retinal disorder including retinitis pigmentosa, advanced glaucoma, degenerative myopia and previous panretinal laser photocoagulation.

CASE 3.6 – 'I have double vision'

A1: What is the differential diagnosis?

- Isolated oculomotor nerve palsy
- Cerebrovascular accident with cranial nerve palsy
- Increased intracranial pressure (ICP)
- Thyroid eye disease (TED)
- Myasthenia gravis
- Multiple sclerosis
- Orbital tumour
- Orbital inflammatory disease (orbital myositis or pseudotumour)
- Trauma (orbital wall fracture)

A2: What issues in the history support the diagnosis?

Diplopia may be caused by a number of possible aetiologies. Monocular diplopia is usually the result of refractive error and/or opacities or irregularities of the optical media, including corneal scarring, cataract, vitreous opacities and macular disturbances. Binocular diplopia may be the presenting symptom of serious underlying neurological, systemic or orbital disease causing misalignment of the visual axes.

Misalignment may be the result of an abnormality of muscle innervation, muscle function or orbital architecture. Ocular motility disorders may result from ischaemic or haemorrhagic brain-stem lesions. There may be involvement of peripheral nerves only, with no central lesion (isolated oculomotor nerve palsy or peripheral mononeuropathy). The pupil may be spared/uninvolved in vasculopathic aetiologies, as the superficial parasympathetic pupillary fibres, which run in the outer aspect of the third nerve, continue to receive a blood supply. This is sometimes referred to as a pupil-sparing or medical third (nerve palsy). Aneurysms of the internal carotid artery (ICA) may develop at the junction with the posterior communicating artery (PCA) or within the cavernous sinus. Aneurysms of the ICA–PCA junction account for a significant proportion (over 50 per cent) of all third cranial nerve palsies, as a result of sudden dilatation of the aneurysm or from subarachnoid haemorrhage. The pupillary fibres are almost invariably affected. This is known as a pupil-involving or surgical third (nerve palsy). However, a significant minority of patients may develop a third cranial nerve palsy due to aneurysmal compression but without pupil involvement. If the diagnosis is unclear, magnetic resonance imaging (MRI) should be performed.

Extraocular muscle involvement is common in patients with dysthyroid eye disease and may be the first sign of the disease. Patients may be hyperthyroid, hypothyroid or euthyroid.

A3: What additional features in the history would you seek to support a particular diagnosis?

It is important to establish whether the diplopia is monocular or binocular. Monocular diplopia disappears when the affected eye is occluded but is still present when the unaffected eye is covered. Binocular diplopia is no longer present when either eye is covered.

Ask about associated symptoms suggestive of intracranial pathology, malignancy or giant cell arteritis such as headache, jaw claudication, scalp tenderness, neck stiffness, weight loss and/or loss of appetite. A detailed headache history must be elicited to determine whether elevated ICP may be present – exacerbating factors such as whether the headache is worse on waking or on bending, lifting, coughing or straining. Is there a history of trauma? Is the diplopia constant or variable (e.g. is it worse towards the end of the day, suggesting an element of fatiguability)?

Determine the meridian of the diplopia – whether the two images are displaced horizontally, vertically or torsionally:

- Horizontal diplopia: the images are 'side by side':
  - Lateral rectus palsy – cranial nerve VI lesion
  - Medial rectus palsy – cranial nerve III lesion or internuclear ophthalmoplegia
- Vertical diplopia: the images are 'one on top of the other':
  - Superior rectus palsy – cranial nerve III lesion
  - Inferior rectus palsy – cranial nerve III lesion
  - Inferior oblique palsy – cranial nerve III lesion
  - Superior oblique palsy – cranial nerve IV lesion
  - TED
  - Orbital floor fracture
- Torsional diplopia: the images are 'tilted':
  - Diplopia is particularly marked in downgaze (e.g. when reading or walking downstairs)
  - Superior oblique palsy – cranial nerve IV lesion

The past medical history is important: diabetes, hypertension, thyroid dysfunction, multiple sclerosis or myasthenia gravis.

A4: What clinical examination would you perform and why?

Inspect the patient for a compensatory head posture. Inspect the eyes for an obvious squint, lid retraction, lid lag on downgaze, exophthalmos/proptosis or enophthalmos (orbital floor fracture). Look for ptosis (cranial nerve III palsy). A full anterior segment examination is necessary. Check the pupils for anisocoria (ipsilateral pupil may be dilated in cranial nerve III palsy) or RAPD, which may indicate optic nerve compression from an orbital lesion (markedly enlarged extraocular muscles in dysthyroid eye disease, orbital tumour, orbital pseudotumour). Examine the extraocular movements for limitation of motility. Check smooth pursuit as well as saccades and convergence. In paralytic strabismus, the diplopia is greatest in the direction of action of the palsied muscle (e.g. a patient with right lateral rectus palsy describes two images having horizontal displacement greatest on looking to the right). However, if there is mechanical restriction of eye movement, the reverse may occur and there may be associated pain on attempted eye movement (e.g. a patient with right inferior rectus restriction [TED or orbital floor fracture] describes vertical diplopia that is greatest in upgaze). It may be possible to tire the muscles, a sign suggestive of myasthenia gravis.

Visual fields to confrontation may demonstrate homonymous hemianopia. Funduscopy may reveal papilloedema or optic atrophy.

Neurological examination may reveal associated pyramidal signs or abnormal movements of the limbs:

- Weber's syndrome: cranial nerve III palsy and contralateral hemiplegia
- Benedikt's syndrome: cranial nerve III palsy with contralateral involuntary movements of the limbs and contralateral hemianaesthesia

- Millard-Gubler syndrome: palsy of cranial nerves VI and VII and contralateral hemiplegia

A5: What investigations would be most helpful and why?

Arteriosclerosis is a common cause of isolated ocular motor palsy in patients aged 60 or over with systemic hypertension. Check the blood pressure. Blood investigations should include FBC, ESR, fasting blood sugar, fasting lipids and/or thyroid function tests depending on clinical findings. Diagnostic investigations of myasthenia gravis should usually include both testing for serum anti-acetylcholine receptor antibodies (binding, blocking and modulating) and repetitive nerve stimulation studies. Single-fibre electromyography is reserved for selected patients in whom other tests have been negative or equivocal. Neuroimaging (computed tomography [CT] and/or MRI) is indicated if intracranial or orbital pathology is suspected.

A6: What treatment options are appropriate?

- Conservative management: relief of diplopia is of major concern to the patient. Temporary prisms incorporated on to the patient's spectacles, or occlusion of one eye, may be necessary until muscle function improves and ocular alignment is re-established. Sometimes permanent prisms are necessary. The patient should be advised to stop driving unless the two images can be aligned.
- Medical treatment: primary treatment of dysthyroid eye disease must include making the patient euthyroid. Corticosteroids and radiotherapy may be necessary if there is keratopathy from corneal exposure or optic nerve compression.
- Many treatment options are available for myasthenia gravis. Initial treatment usually consists of oral pyridostigmine or neostigmine. Systemic prednisolone may be administered together with the anticholinesterase. Azathioprine and plasmapheresis are also effective. Thymectomy in patients with thymoma often results in remission of the disease.
- Surgical treatment: in patients with temporary problems of extraocular muscle innervation or muscle function (e.g. palsy of cranial nerve VI), botulinum toxin may be injected into the overacting antagonist (medial rectus) of the affected muscle (lateral rectus). This induces deliberate temporary paralysis of the medial rectus by chemodenervation until recovery of lateral rectus function occurs.
- Orbital decompression alleviates symptoms and signs of exposure keratopathy or optic nerve compression. Strabismus surgery is sometimes required.

CASE 3.7 – 'I have intermittent loss of vision in one eye for a few seconds and then my vision returns'

A1: What is the differential diagnosis?

Amaurosis fugax (transient visual loss)

A2: What issues in the history support the diagnosis?

Amaurosis fugax is reversible visual obscuration lasting less than 24 hours. It is a subtype of TIA. The blindness or partial blindness usually lasts less than 10 minutes. It may be caused by thromboembolic phenomena, vasospasm, blood hyperviscosity, vasculitis involving blood vessels that supply the visual pathway or intermittent optic nerve compression with gaze-evoked amaurosis. The most common cause of amaurosis fugax is atherosclerosis of the internal carotid or vertebrobasilar system. Amaurosis fugax resulting from involvement of the internal carotid artery system is unilateral.

A3: What additional features in the history would you seek to support a particular diagnosis?

The history is crucial. Visual loss lasting more than 10 minutes or not returning completely should alert one to the possibility of a retinal vascular occlusion. Ask about symptoms of giant cell arteritis such as headache, scalp tenderness, jaw claudication, anorexia and weight loss.

A4: What clinical examination would you perform and why?

Patients should have a thorough examination of the cardiovascular system, including blood pressure, pulse, auscultation for a cardiac murmur and echocardiogram. Auscultate for a carotid bruit, which may indicate carotid artery stenosis from atherosclerosis.

A5: What investigations would be most helpful and why?

An ESR should be requested to exclude possible vasculitis associated with giant cell arteritis, systemic lupus erythematosus (SLE) or other autoimmune disorder. Carotid Doppler ultrasonography will determine the extent of carotid artery stenosis.

A6: What treatment options are appropriate?

After a single TIA, a patient has a risk of stroke at 5 per cent per annum and death at 5 per cent per annum.

- Medical treatment: patients with carotid artery stenosis may be treated with antiplatelet drugs such as aspirin or dipyridamole. Anticoagulation with warfarin may be considered if a cardiac source of recurrent emboli is identified or if the symptoms persist despite antiplatelet drugs.
- Surgical treatment: the role of carotid endarterectomy after a TIA has been the subject of much research. Patients should be referred to a vascular surgeon if carotid endarterectomy is indicated.

CASE 3.8 – 'I have intermittent loss of vision in both eyes and then my vision clears'

A1: What is the differential diagnosis?

- Migraine
- Increased ICP
- Pseudotumour cerebri (idiopathic intracranial hypertension)
- Amaurosis fugax

A2: What issues in the history support the diagnosis?

Migraine is a common cause of visual disturbances in young patients. External compression of blood vessels supplying the visual pathway may also cause transient visual loss. In patients with papilloedema, pressure on blood vessels within the swollen optic nerve head may cause transient loss of vision in one or both eyes. Amaurosis fugax resulting from involvement of the vertebrobasilar system may produce binocular visual obscuration. Episodes usually last less than 1 minute.

A3: What additional features in the history would you seek to support a particular diagnosis?

Establish whether or not the patient has transient visual loss with scintillating scotomata or fortification spectra (coloured zig-zag lines oscillating in brightness) usually lasting 15 to 20 minutes but can last as long as 1 hour. If so, the diagnosis of migraine is very likely. A personal history or family history of migraine is helpful. Determine the nature of the headache, including exacerbating and relieving factors. Raised ICP often causes headache that is worse on waking and exacerbated by bending, straining and coughing. Is there a history of head trauma? Does the headache follow the visual disturbance?

The drug history is important. Tetracycline, steroid use or withdrawal, nalidixic acid, nitrofurantoin, danazol, ciclosporin and vitamin A in excessive doses are all associated with pseudotumour cerebri. Obesity is also a risk factor.

A4: What clinical examination would you perform and why?

Measure visual acuity. Check for an RAPD. Funduscopy may reveal papilloedema or optic atrophy. In patients with migraine, ophthalmic examination and pupillary reflexes are usually normal. Patients simulating visual deficiency always have a normal examination.

A5: What investigations would be most helpful and why?

Request FBC and ESR to exclude anaemia and possible autoimmune disorder or hyperviscosity syndrome. Visual field analysis may detect enlargement of the blind spot. Neuroimaging (CT and/or MRI) may be indicated to exclude a space-occupying lesion, hydrocephalus or dural sinus thrombosis. In patients with pseudotumour cerebri, the cerebrospinal fluid (CSF) opening pressure may be elevated (>200 mmH$_2$O) on lumbar puncture and CSF composition is normal. Lumbar puncture should always be performed with extreme caution in patients with papilloedema.

A6: What treatment options are appropriate?

- Conservative management: pseudotumour cerebri often recovers spontaneously in 3 to 9 months. In patients with dural sinus thrombosis, the thrombosed intracranial venous sinus usually recanalizes with resolution of the pseudotumour cerebri. Weight loss in obese patients may hasten resolution.
- Medical treatment: in patients with pseudotumour cerebri and persisting headache and/or progressive visual loss, acetazolamide (4 g daily) has been shown to decrease ICP. The administration of oral steroids decreases ICP and promotes the resolution of papilloedema.
- The treatment of migraine involves treatment of the acute attack (analgesics and anti-emetics) and prevention of recurrence (β blockers and calcium channel blockers). Prophylactic treatment should be considered in patients with frequent or severe attacks because migraine may rarely be complicated by permanent visual loss or other neurological dysfunction.
- Autoimmune disorders such as SLE need referral to a specialist physician for immunosuppression.
- Surgical treatment: occasionally, lumboperitoneal shunts or optic nerve sheath decompression may become necessary in patients with pseudotumour cerebri.

REVISION PANEL

- Monocular diplopia and binocular diplopia are two distinct entities with different differential diagnoses. Monocular diplopia is usually the result of refractive error and/or opacities or irregularities of the optical media. Binocular diplopia is caused by misalignment of the visual axes.
- Monocular diplopia resolves when the affected eye is covered, but is still present when the unaffected eye is occluded. Binocular diplopia resolves when either eye is covered.
- Aneurysms of the ICA-PCA junction account for a significant proportion of all CN III palsies. An acute painful CN III palsy involving the pupil may be a sign of an expanding aneurysm or subarachnoid haemorrhage and is a neurosurgical emergency.
- A significant minority of patients may develop a third cranial nerve palsy due to aneurysmal compression but without involvement of the pupil.
- Neuroimaging is indicated if intracranial or orbital pathology is suspected.
- Amaurosis fugax is a reversible visual obscuration lasting less than 24 hours. Complete cardiovascular workup is required.
- The most common cause of amaurosis fugax is thromboembolic disease secondary to atherosclerosis of the internal carotid or vertebrobasilar system.
- Other causes of amaurosis fugax include vasospasm, blood hyperviscosity, vasculitis and optic nerve compression.
- Bilateral transient visual loss accompanied by scintillating scotomata or fortification spectra is typical of migraine.
- Elevated intracranial pressure may cause transient visual obscurations in one or both eyes.
- Both migraine and increased intracranial pressure are characterized by headache. The nature of the headache is therefore extremely important in the differential diagnosis.

CASE 3.9 – 'My child's eye has a turn'

A1: What is the differential diagnosis?

- Non-paralytic squint
- Paralytic squint
- Retinoblastoma

A2: What issues in the history support the diagnosis?

Squint or strabismus occurs in about 3 per cent of children. Most cases present between the ages of 3 months and 4 years. Most childhood squints are non-paralytic, but paralytic squints may occur. Exclusion of underlying ocular, orbital and/or systemic disease is of the utmost importance.

A3: What additional features in the history would you seek to support a particular diagnosis?

The antenatal, perinatal and neonatal history, including history of prematurity, birth weight, birth trauma and developmental milestones, is important. Ask about any family history of refractive errors, amblyopia ('lazy eye'), squint, congenital cataract or retinoblastoma. Is there any previous history of occlusion therapy (patching) of one eye, or squint surgery in the child? Are there any associated neurological symptoms – headache, clumsiness, drowsiness or vomiting?

A4: What clinical examination would you perform and why?

Inspect the child for an abnormal head posture, dysmorphic features or hydrocephalus. Examination of the red reflex is extremely important. The red reflex is reduced or absent in cataract or corneal opacification. There may be leukocoria (white pupil) in cataract, retinoblastoma or other posterior segment pathology. Examine extraocular movements for limitation of eye movements indicative of paresis or palsy of a rectus muscle. In children with convergent squints, full abduction of each eye must be demonstrated to ensure that a cranial nerve VI palsy is not present. Dilated funduscopy is essential because conditions such as retinoblastoma may present with strabismus.

A5: What investigations would be most helpful and why?

Cycloplegic refraction with cyclopentolate 0.5 or 1 per cent or atropine 0.1, 0.5 or 1 per cent is mandatory. Ultrasound examination of the posterior segment is performed in cases of media opacity. In some cases CT and/or MRI of the brain, eye and orbit may be indicated.

A6: What treatment options are appropriate?

There is a very close relationship between visual function and ocular alignment in children, and many children with squint develop amblyopia.

- Conservative management: detection and treatment of refractive errors (spectacles) and amblyopia (occlusion therapy of the 'good eye') are important.
- Surgical treatment: ocular realignment by means of strabismus surgery can then be carried out if necessary.
- Retinoblastoma may be treated by chemoreduction and focal therapy (laser photocoagulation and cryotherapy). In some cases, external beam radiotherapy is also needed. Unfortunately, many eyes with advanced disease need to be enucleated.

CASE 3.10 – 'My baby has watery eyes'

A1: What is the differential diagnosis?

- Congenital nasolacrimal duct obstruction
- Congenital glaucoma

A2: What issues in the history support the diagnosis?

The most common cause of watery eyes in the first year of life is congenital obstruction of the nasolacrimal duct (Figure 3.5), caused by failure of canalization of its lower end. Abnormalities of facial bone structure may result in dacryostenosis. However, the most significant cause of watery eyes in neonates and infants is congenital glaucoma. In newborns and very young infants and children, large watery eyes associated with photophobia may be signs of congenital glaucoma.

A3: What additional features in the history would you seek to support a particular diagnosis?

The perinatal history is important to exclude a history of birth trauma or forceps delivery. Enquire whether the watering is associated with photophobia and worse in bright lights. Have the parents noticed enlargement of their child's eye(s)? Is there a sticky mucopurulent discharge suggestive of conjunctivitis?

A4: What clinical examination would you perform and why?

Press on the area over the lacrimal sac (see Figure 3.5) and look for regurgitation of mucoid or mucopurulent fluid. This is typical of nasolacrimal duct obstruction. Important signs of congenital glaucoma include enlargement of the eye(s) and corneal opacification. Dilated funduscopy is essential to exclude posterior segment pathology. Cycloplegic refraction should be performed to detect myopia, which may develop as a result of enlargement of the eye(s).

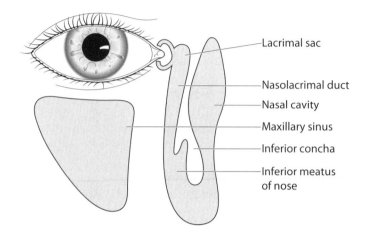

Figure 3.5 Nasolacrimal duct – tear drainage apparatus.

A5: What investigations would be most helpful and why?

Examination under general anaesthesia may be necessary to check intraocular pressures, to measure corneal diameters and to perform detailed retinal examination.

A6: What treatment options are appropriate?

- Conservative management: delayed canalization occurs in 90 per cent of infants by the first birthday, and any surgical intervention should therefore be postponed until then. Daily massage of the lacrimal sac will prevent accumulation of debris and may reduce the risk of dacryocystitis.
- Surgical treatment: if recanalization does not occur and surgery becomes necessary, a syringe and probe of the nasolacrimal duct are performed under general anaesthetic. Sometimes this needs to be repeated. Rarely, intubation of the duct or dacryocystorhinostomy (DCR) is necessary.
- Congenital glaucoma is very rare and should be managed in specialist centres. Surgical intervention is necessary to achieve successful lowering of the intraocular pressure.

REVISION PANEL

- Most childhood squints are non-paralytic, but paralytic squints can and do occur in childhood.
- All children with squint must have dilated funduscopy to exclude retinoblastoma which may present with strabismus.
- Many children with squint develop amblyopia.
- Cycloplegic refraction to detect refractive error is mandatory.
- The most common cause of watery eye(s) in the first year of life is congenital nasolacrimal duct obstruction.
- The most significant cause of watery eye(s) in neonates and infants is congenital glaucoma.

OSCE Counselling cases

OSCE COUNSELLING CASE 3.1 – 'Why am I having difficulty reading since having my cataract surgery?'

Cataract surgery leaves the patient presbyopic. There is loss of unaided near vision.

Normally, the lens of the eye changes shape to focus light onto the retina. The ciliary muscle, which is attached to the lens by the zonules, contracts or relaxes to change the shape of the natural crystalline lens, depending on whether the object being viewed is close or far away. The near reflex consists of ciliary muscle contraction (accommodation), convergence and pupillary constriction.

The natural lens becomes cloudy with age and forms a cataract. This natural lens is removed at the time of cataract surgery and replaced with a synthetic lens implant. The lens implant is usually monofocal in design and also cannot change shape in the same way that the natural lens can. As a result, depending on the power of lens implant chosen, light is focused to form a clear image on the retina for either a distant or a near object, but not for both. So, if vision is very clear for distance, it cannot also be clear for close-up. Increasingly, multifocal implants (rather than monofocal ones) are being used to eliminate this problem, but careful patient selection is advised.

The loss of close-up focusing can be corrected by wearing spectacles or a contact lens. Reading spectacles help to focus clearly on objects that are close, such as small print in a book or newspaper. Reading spectacles may be obtained as a separate pair, or incorporated into bifocals, trifocals or varifocals (also known as progressives).

If the cataract in the other eye needs to be operated on, a lens implant can be chosen that allows good near vision with that eye. The dominant eye is then used for far vision and the non-dominant eye for close vision. This is called monovision. However, this difference in focusing power between the two eyes is sometimes not well tolerated.

OSCE COUNSELLING CASE 3.2 – 'Why can't I see as well now as I did after my cataract surgery 18 months ago?'

During a cataract operation, a clear lens implant is placed inside the eye to replace the natural lens that has become cloudy, forming a cataract. The natural lens is encased in a clear capsular bag. The lens implant is placed 'in the bag', which provides support. The implant sits in the same anatomical position as the natural lens that it has replaced.

In some patients, months or years after cataract surgery the capsule thickens up and becomes cloudy. This is not another cataract, although the symptoms may be the same. It is treated quickly and painlessly in the clinic by using a Nd:YAG laser to make a small hole in the capsule.

Only a small hole is needed, so the lens implant still has plenty of support. This small opening allows light to pass into the eye so that the patient sees clearly again.

REVISION PANEL

- Patients become presbyopic following cataract extraction with (monofocal) intraocular lens implant. The lens implant chosen usually results in clear distance vision, but poor unaided near vision.
- The loss of close-up focusing can be corrected by wearing spectacles or contact lenses. Alternatively, a multifocal intraocular lens implant may be used in suitable cases.
- Monovision is the deliberate placement of a (monofocal) lens implant set for clear distance vision in the dominant eye, and for clear near vision in the non-dominant eye. This may obviate the need for spectacles or contact lenses post-operatively.
- During cataract surgery, the intraocular lens (IOL) implant is placed 'in the bag' to provide capsular support for the IOL.
- In some patients, months or years after cataract surgery, the capsular bag thickens and becomes cloudy.
- The Nd:YAG laser is used to make a small central opening in the capsular bag (capsulotomy), so that the patient sees clearly again.

OSCE COUNSELLING CASE 3.3 – 'Why am I short of breath since starting treatment for glaucoma?'

Timolol is a β-adrenergic blocking agent. It has several potential cardiovascular, respiratory and central nervous system side effects after ocular administration. Patients who are receiving topical ophthalmic timolol should be counselled about and observed for potential side effects.

Cardiovascular

- Bradycardia
- Arrhythmia
- Heart block
- Palpitation
- Cardiac failure
- Pulmonary oedema
- Cardiac arrest
- Hypotension
- Syncope
- Cerebral ischaemia
- Cerebrovascular accident
- Raynaud's phenomenon

Respiratory

- Bronchospasm (predominantly in patients with pre-existing asthma or other bronchial disease)
- Respiratory failure
- Dyspnoea
- Cough

Central nervous system/psychiatric

- Depression
- Somnolence
- Insomnia
- Nightmares

- Hallucinations
- Confusion
- Disorientation
- Anxiety
- Nervousness
- Memory loss

Endocrine

- Masked symptoms of hypoglycaemia in patients with diabetes

Other

- Nausea
- Diarrhoea
- Anorexia
- Dry mouth
- Fatigue
- Impotence.

Note that these potential side effects may be amplified by concomitant use of oral β-blocker treatment.

OSCE COUNSELLING CASE 3.4 – 'I have recently been diagnosed with glaucoma. Can I still drive?'

Update

The Motor Vehicles (Driving Licenses) (Amendment) Regulations 2013 came into force on 8 March 2013. These regulations implement the minimum standards of medical fitness required for eyesight and epilepsy and state:

(1) Impairment of vision is prescribed for the purposes of section 92(2) of the Traffic Act as a relevant disability in relation to an applicant for, or a holder of, a Group 1 license, who is unable to satisfy the following standards—
   (a) the Group 1 visual acuity standard in paragraph (1A);
   (b) the Group 1 visual field standard in paragraph (1C); and
   (c) in the case of a person with diplopia or sight in only one eye, the adaptation standard in paragraph (1D).

(1A) The Group 1 visual acuity standard is—
   (a) a visual acuity of at least 6/12 (decimal 0.5); and
   (b) the ability to read in good daylight a registration mark which is affixed to a motor vehicle and contains characters of the prescribed size, in either case with corrective lenses if necessary.

(1B) For the purposes of paragraph (1A)(b), "characters of the prescribed size" means characters 79 millimetres high and 50 millimetres wide in a case where they are viewed from a distance of—
   (a) 12 metres, by an applicant for, or the holder of, a license authorising the driving of a vehicle of a class included in category K, and
   (b) 20 metres, in any other case.

(1C) The Group 1 visual field standard is—
   (a) a measurement of at least 120 degrees on the horizontal plane;
   (b) an extension of at least 50 degrees left and an extension of at least 50 degrees right;

    (c) an extension of at least 20 degrees above and an extension of at least 20 degrees below the horizontal plane; and

    (d) no significant defects present within a radius of the central 20 degrees.

(1D) The adaptation standard for a person having diplopia or sight in only one eye is that since developing that condition, there has been—

    (a) an appropriate period of adaptation; and

    (b) clinical confirmation of full adaptation.

Note that the eyesight requirements for Group 2 (lorry/bus drivers) are more stringent and that poor night vision may also disqualify a patient from driving. In addition, eyesight complications affecting visual acuity or visual fields are not the only contraindications for driving. Other conditions include, under certain conditions, epileptic seizures, loss of consciousness, TIAs, stroke, angina, myocardial infarction, arrhythmia, syncope, frequent diabetic hypoglycaemic episodes, panretinal laser photocoagulation, drug misuse and dependency, alcohol misuse/dependency and impairment of cognitive function.

    Advice on fitness to drive should be given or considered at every consultation and can be obtained from the medical advisers at the Driver and Vehicle Licensing Agency (DVLA). However, it is the responsibility of the driver to ensure that he or she is in control of the vehicle at all times.

REVISION PANEL

- Topical ophthalmic timolol is a β-adrenergic blocker used in the management of glaucoma.
- Timolol has several potential cardiovascular, respiratory and central nervous system side effects after ocular administration, including among others, bradycardia, heart block, cardiac failure, bronchospasm, depression and memory loss.
- These potential side effects may be amplified by concomitant use of oral β-adrenergic blockers.
- Advice on fitness to drive should be given or considered at every consultation.
- Conditions which affect visual acuity and visual fields may result in patients being unable to meet legal eyesight requirements for driving.
- Poor night driving may also disqualify a patient from driving.
- Other contraindications for driving include, under certain conditions, epileptic seizures, loss of consciousness, stroke, angina, myocardial infarction, arrhythmia, syncope, frequent diabetic hypoglycaemic episodes, panretinal laser photocoagulation, drug or alcohol misuse/dependency and impaired cognitive function.

OSCE COUNSELLING CASE 3.5 – **'I have well-controlled diabetes. I have no problems with my vision. I had my eyes checked 1 year ago. When should I next have my eyes examined?'**

Diabetic retinopathy is the most common cause of blindness in middle-aged people in the United Kingdom. Blindness can often be prevented by early detection and treatment. Diabetic retinopathy may be asymptomatic. This is why at least an annual dilated funduscopy is suggested by the World Health Organization and Diabetes UK. Screening is undertaken to detect disease of any severity and/or to detect disease of sufficient severity to warrant treatment.

    All people with diabetes are at risk of retinopathy, even those whose hyperglycaemia is well controlled. However, the following are some factors that increase the risk of developing retinopathy:

- Duration of diabetes
- Poor glycaemic control
- Hypertension

- Hyperlipidaemia
- Nephropathy (microalbuminuria, proteinuria, renal failure)
- Obesity
- Pregnancy

OSCE COUNSELLING CASE 3.6 – 'Will laser treatment make my vision worse? My neighbour, who also has diabetes, is now blind following laser treatment'

Diabetic retinopathy may be non-proliferative or proliferative. Non-proliferative retinopathy may be mild, moderate or severe. Severe non-proliferative diabetic retinopathy is also known as pre-proliferative retinopathy. Proliferative retinopathy can lead to vitreous haemorrhage and traction retinal detachment. Some patients develop diabetic maculopathy, with oedema and hard exudates at the macula, and/ or macular ischaemia. Several randomized controlled studies have confirmed the effectiveness of laser treatment for high-risk proliferative retinopathy or clinically significant macular oedema.

Laser is a high-energy beam of light that is focused on the retina, thereby inducing thermal damage – laser photocoagulation. Laser treatment has vastly improved the management of diabetic eye disease. However, there are potential complications following all forms of laser surgery. The treatment is given as an outpatient procedure and is usually painless, although some patients experience significant pain and headache. Macular oedema may occur after panretinal laser, especially if the patient has significant renal impairment. This may cause temporary worsening of vision. There is also a risk of permanent reduction in visual fields and night vision after panretinal photocoagulation. Sometimes vision continues to deteriorate despite laser surgery. Visual outcome depends on the severity of the retinopathy and the indication for the laser. The patient may have proliferative retinopathy, diabetic macular oedema that is focal or diffuse, ischaemic maculopathy or a combination of these. The aim of laser surgery is mainly to stabilize vision and prevent progressive visual loss. Vision may not necessarily improve. Each patient is different and every eye reacts differently to laser.

Paracentral scotomata may occur after macular laser treatment and in some centres has been replaced by intravitreal injections of anti-VEGF. There are no licensed VEGF inhibitors for the treatment of non-AMD eye conditions such as proliferative diabetic retinopathy and diabetic macular oedema. Although not licensed as a treatment for eye conditions, Bevacizumab (Avastin) is administered 'off label' in some hospitals in the United Kingdom as an intravitreal injection to treat eye conditions where there are no licensed treatments.

REVISION PANEL

- All patients with diabetes are at risk of diabetic retinopathy, even those whose hyperglycaemia is well controlled.
- Screening detects unrecognized, symptomless, sight-threatening diabetic eye disease.
- At least once per annum fundus examination is recommended for all patients with diabetes. This usually entails dilated funduscopy, but some centres offer photographic retinal screening.
- Several randomized, controlled clinical trials have confirmed the effectiveness of laser treatment for high-risk proliferative retinopathy or clinically significant macular oedema.
- Sometimes vision continues to deteriorate despite laser surgery.
- Although not licensed as a treatment for eye conditions, Bevacizumab (Avastin) is administered 'off label' in some hospitals in the United Kingdom as an intravitreal injection for the treatment of non-AMD eye conditions such as diabetic macular oedema, where there are no licensed treatments.

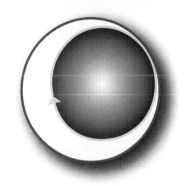

4 Trauma and orthopaedic surgery

Nicole Abdul, Terence McLoughlin

THE PAINFUL HIP

FRACTURES

BACK PROBLEMS

THE PAINFUL HIP

Questions

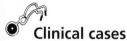
Clinical cases

For each of the clinical case scenarios given

> **Q1:** What is the likely differential diagnosis?
> **Q2:** What issues in the given history support the diagnosis?
> **Q3:** What additional features in the history would you seek to support a particular diagnosis?
> **Q4:** What clinical examination would you perform and why?
> **Q5:** What investigations would be most helpful and why?
> **Q6:** What treatment options are appropriate?

CASE 4.1 – **The toddler who will not weight bear**

A 15-month-old toddler is referred via the general practitioner (GP) because he is refusing to put his right foot down to the ground and walk. Attempts to encourage him to weight bear clearly distress him but, when left to his own devices, although he is slightly off his food and rather unwell, in general terms he will sit and play quietly.

CASE 4.2 – **The boy whose knee hurts and who limps after playing football**

A 9-year-old boy is referred with a 3-month history of knee pain, which seems to be related to him playing football or riding his bike. He can usually do the activity for a short time, but then complains of a painful knee and develops a limp. This lasts for a couple of days before resolving. The next time he plays football or rides his bike the same thing happens.

CASE 4.3 – **The teenager with a groin strain**

A 14-year-old girl who is a little overweight presents with what appears to be a groin strain. She is not a keen athlete but was taking part in games doing the triple jump. She experienced pain in the groin 6 weeks ago and this has not got any better. She has been able to weight bear, but reluctantly, and certainly cannot run.

CASE 4.4 – **A stiff painful hip in a retired man**

A retired man is referred with a 5-year history of increasing pain and stiffness in his right hip. This has gradually got worse and is no longer responding to simple analgesics.

👫 OSCE Counselling cases

OSCE COUNSELLING CASE 4.1 – **'Doctor, I had my hip replaced 2 months ago; it doesn't hurt but I'm still limping'**

OSCE COUNSELLING CASE 4.2 – **'My knee has been hurting for 2 years. I have had two steroid injections in the last year. Does it mean I need to have my knee replaced?'**

Key concepts

THE SURGICAL SIEVE

- Orthopaedics lends itself very well to considering disease types in terms of a surgical sieve. Conditions may be genetic/congenital in origin, developmental, traumatic, inflammatory, infective, neoplastic or degenerative.
- Patients in infancy or early childhood are, naturally, more likely to present with problems related to congenital/genetic or developmental abnormalities. As a result of their immature immune status, they are also more likely to have infective problems. Similarly, they could also present with neoplastic problems.
- Trauma in terms of straightforward isolated limb injuries increases as children become more active and independent. Injuries peak in the form of severe life-threatening multiple trauma in early adult life. Trauma then becomes less common until the effects of osteoporosis and general infirmity supervene, with patients having falls in what would otherwise be fairly safe surroundings, sustaining fractures of pathologically weakened bones.

Answers

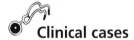

Clinical cases

CASE 4.1 – The toddler who will not weight bear

A1: What is the likely differential diagnosis?

- Transient synovitis of the hip joint (the archetypal cause of irritable hip)
- Septic arthritis of the hip (an acute surgical emergency)
- Osteomyelitis of the proximal femur or pelvis
- Greenstick fracture elsewhere in the right lower limb
- Neoplasia (exceedingly rare)

A2: What issues in the given history support the diagnosis?

Irritable hip is the name given to this type of presentation, but it is not a diagnosis. Think of it as a general term for presentation, such as acute abdomen. Transient synovitis is the most common diagnosis, and is usually seen in children of this age a week or so after an upper respiratory tract infection. It appears to represent a form of cross-reaction between viral antigens and the synovium. It is a self-limiting condition with no adverse sequelae. The child has usually recovered from the upper respiratory tract infection, but occasionally the two things happen concurrently. The child will usually sit comfortably and will be interested in playing, eating etc, but will resist attempts to get him to walk.

A3: What additional features in the history would you seek to support a particular diagnosis?

In septic arthritis the child is usually unwell, off food and wants to lie still. In a classic presentation of a fulminant septic arthritis, even minimal movement will result in extreme pain. In very young children, however, this can be hard to establish, especially if the child is already distressed.

Osteomyelitis usually has a more indolent and less florid presentation, but is invariably seen in a child whose sleep has been disturbed by the pain and who is unwell in other respects.

Greenstick fractures are fairly common in children of this age. A history of the child crying, limping or refusing to weight bear after attempting to kick a football is quite common. The child often twists on the leg supporting the weight, resulting in an undisplaced spiral fracture of the tibia with an intact fibula.

Childhood cancers, although rare, are important not to miss and must be considered as a differential diagnosis in a child refusing to weight bear. Osteosarcoma and Ewing's sarcoma usually present in the teenage years, although they can present in younger children. Benign tumours are also more common in adolescence but have been included here for completeness. You should be aware of the following benign tumours but a detailed knowledge is not expected at an undergraduate level: osteoid osteoma, osteochondroma, chondroblastoma, osteoblastoma, eosinophilic granuloma, fibrous and osteofibrous dysplasia, aneurysmal cysts, unicameral bone cysts and fibromas.

A4: What clinical examination would you perform and why?

A full examination of the child should be performed, checking the temperature, ears, nose and throat in particular. It is often easier to examine the child whilst they are being cuddled by a parent. Examine the normal limb first and tickle the child's toes to see how free the movements are. Then, gently examine the problem limb, starting with a tickle and gentle passive movements, before systematic palpation.

In the child who wishes to lie still, it is worth noting the resting position of the affected limb. To relax the capsule in the presence of an effusion, the hip is instinctively held in a slightly flexed and externally rotated position. In septic arthritis or osteomyelitis, the child is often very unwell and pyrexial. A key feature of septic arthritis is that movement of the limb concerned will be very painful. In other circumstances movement may be possible and usually limited only at the extremes.

Careful clinical examination of the lower limb may reveal localized tenderness in the presence of a greenstick fracture.

Bone tumours present in various ways depending on the pathophysiology. Whilst some may be predominately asymptomatic, others may present with masses, malaise, pain, weight loss, fever and erythema.

A5: What investigations would be most helpful and why?

The most important diagnosis to exclude is that of septic arthritis. A blood sample should be taken for full blood count (FBC), erythrocyte sedimentation rate (ESR) and C-reactive protein (CRP). These are usually normal in transient sympathetic synovitis. If the child is pyrexial, blood cultures should also be taken at this point.

A plain radiograph of the pelvis should be taken. Subtle changes in the soft tissues around the hip may suggest the presence of an effusion in the hip. Osteomyelitis can occasionally be diagnosed from a radiograph although magnetic resonance imaging (MRI) is often needed.

The investigation of choice is that of ultrasonography, which, in skilled hands, readily demonstrates the presence of an effusion; in a cooperative child this can be aspirated.

After careful palpation, radiographs of the area of tenderness will show the presence or absence of a fracture.

The different bone tumours listed above will often produce characteristic abnormalities on radiograph, so it is important to check the films for signs such as radiolucency, bone destruction or atypical bone formation/re-modelling. If these signs are identified it may be necessary to further investigate the lesion with MRI, computed tomography (CT) scanning, and/or biopsy.

A6: What treatment options are appropriate?

Transient sympathetic synovitis requires no specific treatment. It usually resolves in 48 to 72 hours and has no long-term sequelae. Simple analgesia and reassurance are all that is required.

Septic arthritis is an acute surgical emergency. Blood cultures should be obtained before emergency surgery to washout the hip joint. The approach to the hip is a matter of surgical preference. In a well-established septic arthritis, sometimes a repeated washout may be required in order to bring an acute suppurative infection under control.

Systemic antibiotics should ideally be commenced once either an aspiration has been performed or surgical specimens are obtained in the operating theatre. If a child is septic and unwell they may have to be commenced before either of these is performed.

Greenstick fractures in the lower limb are relatively common in toddlers. Plaster of Paris or lightweight polymer cast splintage of the limb is all that is required, and children invariably try to walk on them as soon as the acute pain has resolved. This usually happens within a few days of injury. Plaster immobilization is normally needed for about 3 weeks.

For osteomyelitis, initial radiographs may be entirely unremarkable and MRI or a bone scan may be required to confirm the diagnosis. If diagnosed early enough, antibiotics may be sufficient to obtain resolution. However, once a sequestrum has formed surgical drainage of this is mandatory.

In the rare instance of neoplasm presenting as an irritable hip, the treatment is naturally directed towards identifying and treating the cause. Treatment may range from surgery to chemotherapy/radiotherapy. Benign tumours are often treated with surgery or steroid injections, but treatment is dependent on the type of bone tumour present. At an undergraduate level only a basic knowledge of malignant and benign bone tumours is expected.

CASE 4.2 – **The boy whose knee hurts and who limps after playing football**

A1: What is the likely differential diagnosis?

- Perthes' disease
- Transient synovitis of the hip joint (the archetypal cause of irritable hip)
- Septic arthritis of the hip (an acute surgical emergency)
- Osteomyelitis of the proximal femur or pelvis
- Greenstick fracture elsewhere in the right lower limb
- Metastatic neoplasm (exceedingly rare)

A2: What issues in the given history support the diagnosis?

Perthes' disease is more common in boys and usually presents at school age. Although the disease manifests in the hip it commonly presents with referred pain in the thigh or knee. The child is invariably well and otherwise active but has pain provoked by normal childhood activities.

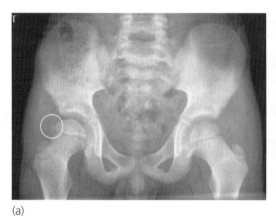
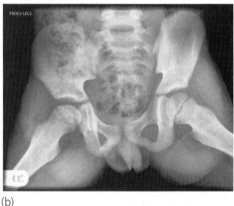

(a)   (b)

Figure 4.1 Perthes' disease. (a) Anteroposterior (AP) and (b) frog lateral views of the pelvis are shown. Apart from a small island of calcification lateral to the femoral head (encircled in [a]), the AP view is relatively normal. The frog lateral view shows collapse of the anterior part of the femoral head.

A3: What additional features in the history would you seek to support a particular diagnosis?

A family history of Perthes' disease strongly supports the diagnosis.

A4: What clinical examination would you perform and why?

The child should be carefully examined from the lumbar spine to the toes. If able to weight bear, a child with Perthes' disease will invariably walk with a limp and an externally rotated leg on the affected side. All movements of the hip will be greatly reduced and painful, particularly internal rotation. A limb length discrepancy may be noted and muscle atrophy might also be present.

A5: What investigations would be most helpful and why?

Plain radiographs, (anteroposterior (AP) pelvis and frog lateral) should be performed. Depending on the stage or grade (severity) of the disease, the femoral epiphysis may show cystic or sclerotic changes. There may be a subchondral fracture giving a 'head-within-a-head' appearance. The femoral head may show 'at-risk' signs, indicating deformation, with flattening of the head. The hip is therefore at risk of changing from a ball-and-socket joint into a hinge one. In cases of doubt these can be supplemented with either a bone scan or preferably MRI.

A6: What treatment options are appropriate?

The goal of treatment in Perthes' disease is to ensure that the child achieves skeletal maturity with a round femoral head in a round hip socket.

The disease has been characterized as an osteochondritis. It is a rather enigmatic condition and, for reasons that are poorly understood, part of the femoral epiphysis or growth centre undergo avascular necrosis. This naturally leads to softening and potential deformation of the femoral head. The younger the child at presentation and being of male sex are associated with a better prognosis.

In milder cases of the disease, treatment might not be needed and non-weight-bearing exercises such as swimming may be encouraged. In more severe forms of the disease, treatment may involve osteotomy of the proximal femur or the acetabulum; confining the child to a cast until the phases of softening, deformation, healing and consolidation of the femoral head have run their course; physiotherapy; or bed rest and crutches.

CASE 4.3 – **The teenager with a groin strain**

A1: What is the likely differential diagnosis?

The probable diagnosis is a slipped upper femoral epiphysis (SUFE). This is also known as slipped capital femoral epiphysis.

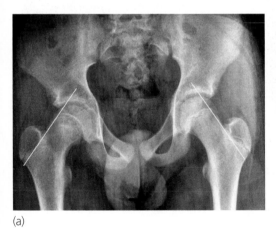
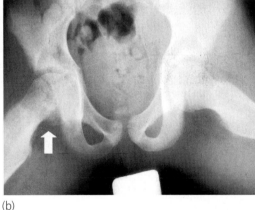

(a)   (b)

Figure 4.2 Slipped upper femoral epiphysis. (a) The anteroposterior pelvis radiograph shows little apart from the subtle sign that a line drawn on the lateral aspect of the asymptomatic femoral neck just passes through the edge of the femoral head. When drawn on the symptomatic side, the line misses the femoral head altogether. (b) As the femoral head slips posteriorly, the displacement is best seen on the frog lateral view. As this is a chronic slip, new bone has formed at the posterior margin of the femoral neck in an effort to shore up the femoral head (arrow).

A2: What issues in the given history support the diagnosis?

The history given is a typical presentation. Pitfalls in the typical presentation are that there might be no associated traumatic event and, as in Perthes' disease, the pain can be manifest in the thigh or knee.

A3: What additional features in the history would you seek to support a particular diagnosis?

The incidence of bilateral slip is about 20 per cent and occasionally there is also a family history. Risk factors for the disease include obesity, endocrine disorders such as hypopituitarism/hypothyroidism/pseudohypoparathyroidism, and exposure to radiation.

A4: What clinical examination would you perform and why?

If the patient can walk, careful evaluation of the gait pattern should be performed, paying attention to external rotation (which may be present constantly), and range of active and passive motion while lying supine. Patients with SUFE will have a reduced range of movement, especially internal rotation and abduction.

A5: What investigations would be most helpful and why?

A plain AP radiograph of the pelvis is essential, and thus must be accompanied by a frog lateral. As the femoral head epiphysis slips posteriorly as well as inferiorly, it is thrown into clear profile only on the radiograph when the frog lateral view is obtained. The plain AP radiograph can look deceptively normal even in the presence of a significant slip, which is obvious on a frog lateral view. An earlier characteristic change on the radiograph is widening of the epiphyseal line.

A6: What treatment options are appropriate?

The child should be admitted and put to bed. The operation of choice is that of fixing the slipped upper femoral epiphysis in situ using percutaneous screws. This prevents further slippage and encourages the physis actually to ossify and close. The screws should be left in place until skeletal maturity.

Slips can be classified into acute or chronic, stable or unstable. Although this case did have an apparent acute precipitating cause, because of the interval between this occurring and the presentation, it would be classified as chronic. As the child can weight bear it is classified as being stable; if the child cannot weight bear, the slip is unstable. In acute slips, which have occurred, for example, in a fall from a bicycle in an otherwise normal hip, efforts to reduce the femoral epiphysis and then fix it are advisable. In chronic slips, because of the rapid nature of remodelling, attempts to effect a reduction are fraught with danger and can lead to avascular necrosis of the femoral head.

CASE 4.4 – A stiff painful hip in the retired man

A1: What is the likely differential diagnosis?

- Osteoarthritis of the hip
- Delayed degenerative presentation of:
  - Developmental hip dysplasia
  - Perthes' disease
  - Slipped capital femoral epiphysis
- Paget's disease
- Metastatic bone disease

A2: What issues in the given history support the diagnosis?

In osteoarthritis the start of pain is typically associated with activity. Stiffness is often worse in the morning and then limbers up with gentle activity. As the day wears on, the pain and stiffness recur.

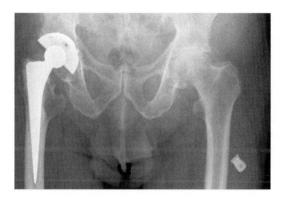

Figure 4.3 A radiograph showing a right total hip replacement in situ.

Simple analgesia and anti-inflammatory drugs are usually of benefit, but as the joint degeneration worsens they invariably become ineffective. It is usually about this point in time that patients start to tolerate the use of a walking aid such as a stick or crutches.

End-stage disease is indicated by pain at night preventing the patient sleeping.

A3: What additional features in the history would you seek to support a particular diagnosis?

The absence of a history of problems in childhood goes strongly against a delayed presentation of a childhood problem. Post-traumatic osteoarthritis does occur as a consequence of acetabular or proximal femoral fractures, but these are rare in the general population. The traumatic episode is usually clearly remembered.

Paget's disease often has a similar presentation to that of osteoarthritis, and can also coexist with it. Along with metastatic bone disease, night pain, unrelated to daytime activity, is more common. The disease is a benign tumour of osteoclasts which results in a dramatic increase in bone turnover. As the new bone is woven, it is softer than its healthy lamellar counterpart; consequently, it may bend or even fracture under normal loads.

Metastatic disease may present in patients who have a known primary (classically prostate, breast, thyroid, kidney, myeloma or lung). Alternatively, the primary may be occult.

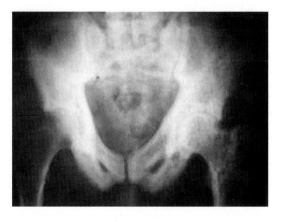

Figure 4.4 A radiograph of a patient with Paget's disease.

A4: What clinical examination would you perform and why?

Careful clinical examination, including evaluation of the limb length, gait pattern, and passive and active movements, is required.

A5: What investigations would be most helpful and why?

Plain radiographs of the pelvis and lateral view of the affected hip will give the diagnosis. The typical radiological features of osteoarthritis are those of loss of joint space, subchondral sclerosis, and cyst and osteophyte formation, with the possibility of a loss of alignment at the joint. As the hip is a ball-and-socket joint this is usually difficult to appreciate.

Paget's disease can affect one bone or many. It may be limited to the proximal femur, ischium, pubis, ilium or the whole innominate bone. The bone is diffusely sclerotic and thickened, and may have areas that look washed out.

The lesion in metastatic disease is usually lytic and, if destruction continues, a pathological fracture can occur. Prostatic metastases cause sclerotic lesions.

A6: What treatment options are appropriate?

The current best available treatment option is a total hip replacement. This is a major operation and consists of replacement of both acetabular and femoral sides of the hip joint. A variety of implants and techniques are available. The technicalities, the choice of which is beyond the scope of this publication, and the long-term results of these are indeed similar. Total hip replacement affords a good range of painless motion and most patients are capable of abandoning walking aids 6 to 12 weeks after surgery. Most arthroplasties last 15 to 20 years before needing revision. Early revision can be needed because of recurrent dislocation or septic loosening.

Skin organisms such as *Staphylococcus aureus/epidermidis* are inevitably introduced into the operative field at the time of surgery. This does not usually cause any problems; however, in a small percentage of patients, infection or a slow loosening process occurs with osteolysis around the implants. Revision surgery in these cases is normally completed as a staged procedure, which appears to carry the least risk of recurrence of infection.

Aseptic loosening occurs much later and seems to be as a result of the body's own response to wear-and-tear debris from the prosthetic components. Currently there is debate about the exact pathophysiology of this process but osteolysis does occur.

In years gone by hip fusion was the mainstay of treatment for patients who would otherwise lead an active life. Patients whose mobility was much more restricted were often treated with excision arthroplasty known as a girdlestone procedure. The femoral head and neck were removed leaving the intertrochanteric area of the femur to articulate with the lateral cortex of the pelvis. This would appear to be a mutilating procedure but it was effective in relieving severe end-stage arthritic pain. Patients were usually able to mobilize with the use of walking aids for distances sufficient for them to be mobile around their own homes.

Paget's disease can usually be managed well with non-operative measures as for osteoarthritis. Bisphosphonates are very effective in managing pain that does not otherwise respond.

In occult malignancy the primary should be sought and treated. Non-steroidal anti-inflammatory drug (NSAID) and/or radiotherapy treatment can be given, if appropriate, to relieve bone pain. Prophylactic stabilization of the bone should be carried out if a fracture is impending.

ṙṙ OSCE Counselling cases

OSCE COUNSELLING CASE 4.1 – 'Doctor, I had my hip replaced 2 months ago; it doesn't hurt but I'm still limping'

Various approaches to the hip for hip replacement surgery have been described. One common approach detaches some of the principal abductors of the hip; although these are repaired at the time of surgery, sometimes the repair fails and the abductors avulse from the greater trochanter. When this occurs the patient normally notices a tearing sensation and there is a sudden dramatic deterioration in physical performance; not only that, but the hip often becomes unstable and can dislocate. Fortunately this particular complication is rare.

It is a little more common for the superior gluteal nerve to be stretched during elevation of the abductor muscles. If this occurs and the nerve does not recover, a permanent abductor lurch or Trendelenburg gait can result. However, more commonly there is post-operative wasting of the same abductor muscles, which recovers with time and mobilization. Specific physiotherapy can sometimes be needed, particularly in patients who are a little more wary of aggressively mobilizing themselves and getting out and about. Simple reassurance and targeted physiotherapy are usually all that is needed.

OSCE COUNSELLING CASE 4.2 – 'My knee has been hurting for 2 years. I have had two steroid injections in the last year. Does it mean I need to have my knee replaced?'

Knee replacement surgery is a very good option to relieve intractable pain from degenerative joint disease. It is a relatively safe and highly successful procedure, which is carried out thousands of times every year in the United Kingdom.

The risks of having serious complications are low but there are no trivial complications from joint replacement surgery. Any problems such as infection, venous thrombosis, or wear of the artificial joint, can lead to potentially disastrous consequences. However 90 per cent of patients have joint replacements that last between 15 and 20 years, and revision surgery is possible (although often difficult) for those cases where infection occurs or the artificial joint wears out.

The indications for joint replacement surgery relate to quality of life. It is a question of balancing the risks of major complications against the benefits of the elimination of pain and restoration of mobility. Patients should be encouraged wherever possible to use simple analgesics or anti-inflammatories if they can tolerate them, to lose weight, use physiotherapy and exercise, and simple walking aids, such as a walking stick, for long distances, to delay the need for joint replacement surgery. It is a better idea for someone to overcome his or her pride and use a walking stick than to risk serious complications from joint replacement surgery. However, many people reach an end stage where, if they have been active during the day, the pain is so bad at night that they cannot sleep. When this is happening regularly, joint revision surgery is a reasonable option.

These similar paradigms hold true for hip replacements.

REVISION PANEL

- Transient synovitis is a common diagnosis in children presenting with a reluctance to weight bear who have recently had a respiratory tract infection.
- Septic arthritis often presents in patients who are very unwell and pyrexial, they may even be septic.
- Greenstick fractures commonly present after trauma and the child will express that he or she is in pain.
- Perthes' disease often presents with pain in the hip or knee. Range of movement will be greatly decreased and the child may have a limp.
- In Perthes' disease the femoral epiphysis undergoes avascular necrosis which leads to deformation of the femoral head.
- Slipped upper femoral epiphysis (SUFE) is common in boys between the ages of 10 and 17 years old.
- Patients with SUFE often have pain in the hip/thigh/knee on physical activities such as running or jumping. They will have a greatly reduced range of motion.
- In SUFE, the proximal growth plate is unstable, causing it to slip either in an acute or chronic setting.
- Paget's disease causes an increase in bone turnover which produces bone that is structurally weak. This can lead to deformation and/or fracture of the affected bones. The bones appear thickened and sclerotic on radiograph.
- The typical radiological features of osteoarthritis are loss of joint space, subchondral sclerosis and cyst and osteophyte formation.
- Most metastatic lesions are lytic but prostatic metastases cause sclerotic lesions.
- Hip surgery can result in damage to muscles, nerves and vessels. Nerve damage can recover, although if permanent may leave the patient with long-term sensory or motor deficiency. Physiotherapy can help to build up muscle strength around the joint post-operatively.

Joint replacement surgery should be delayed, where possible, by treating patients with analgesia and anti-inflammatory drugs (if appropriate), losing weight, physiotherapy or the use of walking aids.

FRACTURES

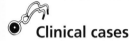

Clinical cases

For each of the clinical case scenarios given

> **Q1:** What is the likely differential diagnosis?
> **Q2:** What issues in the given history support the diagnosis?
> **Q3:** What additional features in the history would you seek to support a particular diagnosis?
> **Q4:** What clinical examination would you perform and why?
> **Q5:** What investigations would be most helpful and why?
> **Q6:** What treatment options are appropriate?

CASE 4.5 – The schoolboy with a femoral shaft fracture

An 8-year-old boy was riding his bike and attempted to do a jump; he fell off the bike landing on an extended right leg, which twisted and gave way beneath him; he has been brought to hospital by ambulance. He is in a great deal of pain and when he cries out you notice that the right femur bends in the middle. The leg is obviously shortened and externally rotated.

CASE 4.6 – The skateboarding teenager with a broken wrist

A 14-year-old girl was skateboarding, fell on to an outstretched left hand and has presented with an obviously deformed left wrist with blunting of sensation in the thumb, index and middle fingers.

CASE 4.7 – The young adult with multiple injuries

A motorcyclist was in collision with a parked van when he attempted to weave in and out of traffic. He has been conscious since the time the ambulance service arrived. He is able to speak and is complaining of pain in the lower abdomen, hips and right lower leg. He has a respiratory rate of 25/min, a heart rate of 120 beats/min and a blood pressure of 90/70 mm Hg. There is obvious tenderness in the suprapubic area and there is a wound over the subcutaneous border of the distal right tibia with bone visible. Q2 is not applicable in this case.

CASE 4.8 – The elderly woman with hip fracture

A 78-year-old woman was being escorted to the bathroom in her residential home when she tripped and fell, injuring her right hip. Her right leg is shortened and externally rotated. She appears fairly comfortable at rest but any attempts at movement or change of position on the bed result in a great deal of pain.

ii OSCE Counselling cases

OSCE COUNSELLING CASE 4.3 – **'Doctor, I have a pin and plate in my leg. Do they need to be removed?'**

OSCE COUNSELLING CASE 4.4 – **'Doctor, with this open fracture of my tibia, am I going to lose my leg?'**

Key concepts

Restoration of function is the goal of treatment. Advances have been made in recent years in refining the management of fractures. The goal is always to restore the patient to normal or as close to normal function as circumstances will allow.

The management of the fracture begins with the evaluation of the patient as a whole. The needs of an 8-year-old child are completely different from those of an 80-year-old adult. Similarly, the range of complications to which each could be subjected is again very different. Broadly speaking, after a thorough clinical examination of the whole patient, followed by that of the affected limb, an obviously dislocated joint or malaligned fracture in which the skin is threatened from pressure within can be realigned, splinted with a plaster of Paris backslab and then evaluated with a radiograph. In cases of uncertainty the radiograph can sometimes be deferred until after the plaster has been applied. It should always be borne in mind that adequate immobilization is the best form of pain relief for a fractured limb.

Children with fractures tolerate bed rest and immobilization in casts much better than adults do. Thus methods can be employed in the management of childrens' fractures that have been surpassed by more active intervention in adult injuries.

If there is a breach in skin continuity over the fracture, it is described as an open fracture. Individual hospitals will usually have a protocol for the management of open fractures that will involve prompt antibiotic administration, tetanus cover, a photograph being taken of the injury and emergency surgery to thoroughly débride and wash out the wound in order to reduce the risk of infection. After evaluation of the soft tissue envelope and establishing of the presence or absence of wounds, and the presence of pulses, sensation and movement in the limb distal to the injury, the radiographs can be evaluated usefully. In the bone, the fracture location (diaphysis or metaphysis) can be identified along with the pattern of the fracture – transverse, oblique, spiral or comminuted. If there are more than two fracture fragments the fracture is comminuted; if there is a soft tissue wound (an open fracture) or nerve or blood vessel injury, the fracture is described as being complicated. It is especially important, if the fracture is in the metaphysis, to decide specifically whether or not it involves the adjacent joint. Similarly, to evaluate an injured limb it should be possible to see the joint both above and below the fracture on the radiograph to exclude other concomitant injuries or fracture extension lines.

If a fracture involves the joint and is displaced, the treatment is to reduce the joint to an anatomical position and hold it rigidly in that position until fracture healing occurs. Other fractures of long bones can be treated well by any method that realigns the limb in terms of length, rotation and angulation, and simply holds it in that position. Fracture union occurs more rapidly in low-energy injuries, which are usually buckle or greenstick fractures in children or spiral fractures in the long bones. Transverse and oblique fractures, those with comminution and also those with overlying soft tissue wounds are high-energy injuries and will require prolonged support to maintain the reduction before union occurs.

Special mention needs to be made of the increasing problems seen in the elderly population suffering the effects of osteoporosis. Fractures of the spine, wrist and proximal femur carry a huge morbidity for the patients who have these injuries. Osteoporotic spinal fractures have no specific management other than prevention. Wrist and hip fractures are common. Hip fractures are usually seen in the more frail elderly population, and the goal of treatment is to restore the patient to mobility as soon as possible after the injuries. If the patient is immobile, surgery is still often the only humane solution because this affords the best and most rapid form of pain relief.

Answers

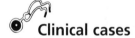

Clinical cases

CASE 4.5 – **The schoolboy with a femoral shaft fracture**

A1: What is the likely differential diagnosis?

The appearances described are those typical for a femoral shaft fracture in a child. As the soft tissues are pliable, alarming deformation can appear in the thigh when the distressed child attempts to move. This not surprisingly increases the pain and worsens the situation.

A2: What issues in the given history support the diagnosis?

The scenario and physical signs described are entirely consistent with sustaining a fracture such as a spiral fracture of the shaft of the femur. This can be confirmed with plain radiographs after adequate splinting (see below).

A3: What additional features in the history would you seek to support a particular diagnosis?

Little more can be obtained from the history.

A4: What clinical examination would you perform and why?

The child should be examined rapidly to exclude any further injuries from which the child is being distracted. Once this has been done a Thomas splint should be applied to the leg, having given the child analgesia and allowing him to be comforted wherever possible by his mother or father. The Thomas splint is applied using skin traction tapes to each side of the leg and the hoop of the splint is slid up the leg, which rests on felt that is attached to the long side bars of the splint to make a cradle. The traction cord is then tied to the end of the splint, and the leg is padded and bandaged to give it further support. This rapidly relieves pain and the limb can be examined for sensation and pulses.

A5: What investigations would be most helpful and why?

Plain AP and lateral radiographs of the femur are required. The hip and knee should be visible on the radiographs and this will allow the fracture to be characterized.

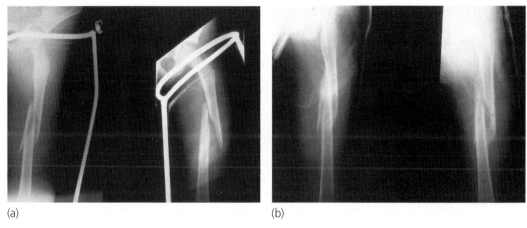

(a)   (b)

Figure 4.5 Closed femoral shaft fracture: (a) anteroposterior (AP) and (b) attempted lateral views of the femur showing a multi-fragmentary (or comminuted) spiral fracture of the femoral shaft at the junction of the upper and middle thirds of the shaft.

A6: What treatment options are appropriate?

For children of this age, provided that the application of skin traction can restore the alignment of the limb and rotation can be controlled by careful readjustment of the traction apparatus, such injuries can be managed very well by closed non-operative means. If non-operative management is planned, balanced traction should be applied with the Thomas splint suspended from Balkan beams attached to the patient's bed. Weekly radiographs are required along with meticulous pressure area care. It is a good idea for the radiographs to be requested at the beginning of the week so any adjustments can be made during the subsequent 5 working days. It is important for the child and the parents to understand that frequent readjustments of one part of the traction or another are necessary until callus forms. Spiral fractures are particularly suitable to be treated in this way because they heal quite rapidly. Alarming fracture gaps between the bone ends in femoral fractures in children are of no real consequence provided that the fracture is not distracted (i.e. pulled apart). Rapid healing will occur and most children can be mobilized after spending 6 to 8 weeks in the Thomas splint. In transverse fractures in which the bone ends are overlapping or in cases where the child has other injuries and is otherwise unsuitable for non-operative management, plating has been carried out successfully in children, which carries a relatively low complication risk. Femoral plating does, however, require the plate to be removed at a later date.

Another alternative is to stabilize the fracture using elastic nails. These are slender metal rods that can be inserted from just proximal to the distal femoral epiphysis. One is inserted on each side and these will act as an elastic splint. For fractures of a highly unstable pattern they are not really suitable. Care should be taken when inserting elastic nails to ensure that they do not go through the growth plate, as this can cause disruption and lead to premature fusion of the plate, affecting growth.

CASE 4.6 – The skateboarding teenager with a broken wrist

A1: What is the likely differential diagnosis?

The differential diagnosis rests between a Salter-Harris type II fracture of the distal radius, the most common injury, a metaphyseal fracture of the distal radius, a fracture of a carpal bone, or more rarely a dislocation of the carpus. The presence of blunting of sensation in the median nerve distribution of the hand suggests an associated neuropraxia of the median nerve.

A2: What issues in the given history support the diagnosis?

Radiological evaluation will determine which fracture is present.

A3: What additional features in the history would you seek to support a particular diagnosis?

Little more can be obtained from the history.

A4: What clinical examination would you perform and why?

The patient should be examined to make sure that there are no other undisclosed injuries. If the arm is very obviously fractured a backslab should be applied and radiographs obtained. Detailed physical examination is required to carefully document the nerve, vessel and soft tissue injuries associated with fractures, as has been done. In the presence of median nerve symptoms rapid reduction of the fracture is required, and this may also warrant stabilization to allow the carpal tunnel to be decompressed acutely. Tenderness in the anatomical snuffbox may indicate a scaphoid fracture.

A5: What investigations would be most helpful and why?

Plain radiographs will give the diagnosis along with the pattern of displacement and allow the patient's fracture management to be planned. Be aware that scaphoid fractures may not be identified on initial radiographs, so the patient may need to return a week later to have a check radiograph if you suspect this diagnosis.

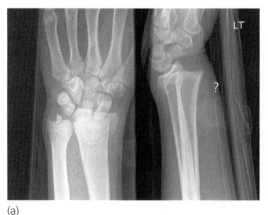 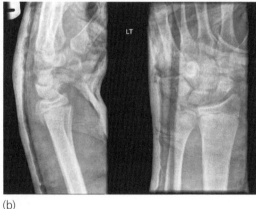

(a) (b)

Figure 4.6 Salter-Harris type II fracture of the distal radius.

A6: What treatment options are appropriate?

Whatever the fracture pattern, in the presence of median nerve symptoms, reduction should be done promptly. In a compliant patient reduction can be attempted with the use of gas and air for pain relief once the pattern of the fracture has been defined. However, if access to the operating theatre can be gained quickly it would be better to take the patient to theatre.

Fractures of the epiphysis or growth area of bone are described using the Salter-Harris classification:

- Type I is a shear fracture in which the whole of the epiphysis is sheared off. This is similar to an acute slip of the capital femoral epiphysis.
- Salter-Harris type II fractures are the most common type. Here the whole of the epiphysis is sheared and the triangle of metaphysis remains attached, which is what is seen at the wrist.

- Type III and type IV fractures both involve a split of the epiphysis. In type III it is the detached split fragment of the epiphysis that displaces with no metaphyseal attachment. In type IV there is a split of the epiphysis with a triangle of metaphysis attached.
- A fifth type has since been described and this is a crush injury to the epiphyseal plate. It is usually a retrospective diagnosis because there is very little to see on the initial radiographs. This is rare.

Accurate reduction of Salter-Harris injuries is required along with adequate stabilization. If there is loss of position beyond 7 days from the original manipulation, further manipulations are believed to carry a risk of partial or complete growth arrest so are unadvisable.

Early reduction is required and this can, as a result of the irregular surface of the epiphysis, require more effort than may first be appreciated, so reduction may have to be done in theatre under general anaesthetic.

Re-examination of the child's hand after immobilization is essential. The simple intervention of applying a backslab and elevating the limb may relieve some of the median nerve symptoms. In a situation in which the median nerve symptoms are improving, acute carpal tunnel decompression is probably not indicated. If the symptoms are worsening the fracture needs to be reduced and held in such a way that the carpal tunnel can be decompressed.

In most circumstances closed reduction and application of a moulded cast are sufficient to retain the reduced position.

Should any further operative intervention be required, insertion of a smooth K-wire (1 or 2) to transfix the metaphyseal fragment to the intact metaphysis is all that is required to stabilize this type of injury; carpal tunnel decompression can then be carried out without difficulty.

It should be borne in mind that, if the symptoms are severe, complete resolution of median nerve problems is not seen despite a rapid decompression. This can take several weeks to resolve.

CASE 4.7 – **The young adult with multiple injuries**

A1: What is the likely differential diagnosis?

The patient is in hypovolaemic shock. The possible reason is an 'open book injury' to the pelvis caused by the motorcycle's fuel tank being pushed into the pelvis. He also clearly has an open fracture of the distal right tibia – a serious injury and one that requires prompt treatment.

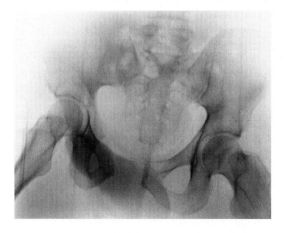

Figure 4.7 'Open book injury' to the pelvis: an external rotation injury (open book injury to the right hemipelvis).

A2: What issues in the given history support the diagnosis?

Not applicable

A3: What additional features in the history would you seek to support a particular diagnosis?

It would be useful to know whether the patient had lost consciousness, if any witnesses are available to question. It is helpful to know whether the patient is covered for tetanus immunization, whether he has any allergies and, as the patient will require emergency surgery, any significant past medical history and when he last ate or drank.

A4: What clinical examination would you perform and why?

The patient has already been evaluated in terms of the primary survey in accordance with Advanced Trauma Life Support (ATLS) protocol. The purpose of the primary survey is to identify and treat immediate life-threatening problems. The airway is evaluated first; the patient who can talk is preserving his own airway, and the one unable to talk must have his airway preserved for him.

Breathing is evaluated next; auscultation and percussion are carried out particularly at the apex and in the base. Bear in mind that the patient is supine and not erect as in a classic physician's chest examination. Therefore air will be present on the anterior chest at the apex and fluid (blood) will collect in the posterior chest, which is the base.

The position of the trachea is checked. All patients should have high-flow oxygen supplied and the cervical spine immobilized in a hard collar. Measurement of heart rate and blood pressure is part of the circulation assessment. Tachycardia (a heart rate of 100 beats/min or more in an adult) is the earliest sign of hypovolaemic shock. Once it is identified a rapid bolus of fluids should be given and the source of haemorrhage sought. Specimens should be sent to the laboratory for cross-matching of six units, and FBC, urea and electrolytes (U&Es), and a clotting screen done. A radiograph of the chest will show any subtle signs of a haemothorax developing, and one of the pelvis is mandatory whether or not the patient has pain.

Depending on the patient's injuries and stability, a 'pan CT scan' may be performed in order to quickly identify the injuries the patient has sustained.

Careful re-evaluation of the patient's response to the fluid bolus is essential. The patient will return to haemodynamic normality and stay there, the tachycardia will return to normal, the pulse pressure will widen or the systolic blood pressure will rise. If the patient remains haemodynamically normal and well perfused with a good urine output, he or she is described as a good responder. Initially, the fluid bolus may produce the benefits, but then when the fluid infusion rate is reduced the patient's observations again decline. This patient would be a transient responder, indicating that the bolus given has not replaced the fluid losses because bleeding is continuing. In these circumstances it is easy to appreciate the importance of identifying the source of potential haemorrhage so this can be dealt with rapidly. The patient whose observations remain unchanged is a non-responder and imminent exsanguination is likely. Emergency surgery is indicated. While waiting for this to become clear, it is possible to extend the patient's examination and ensure that no injuries from which the patient has been distracted are overlooked.

The pelvic injury (an open book) with separation of the symphysis at the front and gaping of the sacroiliac joint at the back should be stabilized by binding the pelvis tightly using a pelvic binder. The hips and knees should be flexed slightly over a rolled-up blanket, with binding around the distal femurs. It is important to bear in mind that the urinary tract, bowel, major blood vessels and nerves are in close proximity to the pelvic bones, so these structures may have been damaged in patients with a pelvic injury. Your examination should include trying to determine whether these injuries are likely or not. Be aware that a large amount of blood can collect in the pelvis, which can lead to hypovolaemic shock. The open fracture of the tibia should be photographed if a camera is available, and the distal neurovascular status assessed. The wound should be covered in an antiseptic-soaked swab and the limb immobilized in a plaster of Paris backslab. This limb should remain entirely covered until the patient is in the operating theatre.

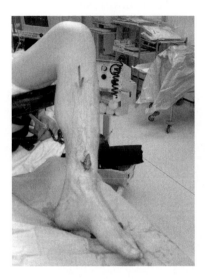

Figure 4.8 Image showing an open fracture of the left distal tibia.

A5: What investigations would be most helpful and why?

If the patient's condition allows, CT may be useful in such circumstances to exclude any serious concomitant injury. However, if the patient is a transient or non-responder emergency surgery is required. Anteroposterior and lateral radiographs of the fractured lower limb will be needed prior to operative management of this injury. Pelvic radiographs will also need to be obtained.

A6: What treatment options are appropriate?

Once the pelvis has been bound some improvement in the patient's haemodynamic status should be seen. A thorough examination should be performed of the patient's urogenital triangle, and any signs of urethral injury, such as blood at the meatus, heavy scrotal bruising or a prostate difficult to feel on rectal examination, should be noted. Do not attempt urethral catheterization in a patient where damage to the urinary tract is suspected.

The patient should be taken to the operating theatre and the pelvis stabilized using an external fixator. If the patient's haemodynamic status does not improve a laparotomy may be required. This may be directed by the findings on CT in a patient who was in a more stable condition.

The open fracture to the tibia should be managed by following the hospital protocol for treating open fractures. This will involve antibiotic administration, tetanus cover, the wound being debrided of all dead, devascularized and foreign tissue, and a thorough washout as an emergency. The tibia should be stabilized using either an external fixator or an intramedullary nail.

Experience shows that soft tissue coverage should be achieved within 5 days of such an injury and, once it is clear that the margins of the soft tissue envelope are viable, definitive bone stabilization should be done as soon as possible.

Experience shows that it is rarely possible to close such wounds primarily and the assistance of a plastic surgeon is required. Local fasciocutaneous rotation flaps, or even free tissue transfers of the latissimus dorsi or rectus abdominis muscles are often required in these circumstances.

CASE 4.8 – **The elderly woman with hip fracture**

A1: What is the likely differential diagnosis?

The differential diagnosis of fracture of the proximal femur may be as follows:

- Intracapsular
- Extracapsular: intertrochanteric or subtrochanteric

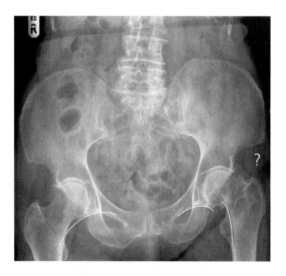

Figure 4.9 A radiograph showing a left intracapsular neck of femur fracture.

A2: What issues in the given history support the diagnosis?

No specific features in the history enable one to differentiate these injuries from each other.

A3: What additional features in the history would you seek to support a particular diagnosis?

Increasing age and being of the female sex are predisposing factors for osteoporosis. Similarly the residents of nursing and residential homes represent a high-risk group within this population.

A4: What clinical examination would you perform and why?

General clinical examination and assessment of the affected limb including neurovascular status

A5: What investigations would be most helpful and why?

Pre-operative work-up of the patient needs to answer the question 'Is this patient as well as possible?' and, if unwell, 'can they be optimized for theatre?' Routine bloods are required. If the patient has a pacemaker it needs to be checked pre-operatively. Electrocardiogram (ECG), chest radiograph and a cross-match of two units of blood are also needed.

A6: What treatment options are appropriate?

Treatment options are tailored to the needs of the individual and the pattern of the fracture. Intracapsular hip fractures are especially problematic when managed by internal fixation. The femoral head has a retrograde blood supply in which the majority of blood vessels supplying it are bound to the femoral neck.

If the neck is fractured and displaced these vessels are interrupted. In common with other bones with a retrograde blood supply (such as the scaphoid), intracapsular fractures of the neck of femur are fraught with problems of avascular necrosis of the femoral head and also non-union.

In young patients, such as motorcyclists, who sustain a high-energy injury resulting in such a fracture, open reduction and internal fixation are mandatory and should be done as early as the patient's general condition permits.

In an elderly patient, who would not be able to mobilize and is non–weight bearing, a better option is to operate, discard the fractured femoral head and neck segment, and replace this with a hemiarthroplasty. A variety of implants are available that may be secured in the femoral shaft using cemented or uncemented methods. Such implants enable the patients to mobilize as soon as pain permits and functional outcome in the population with restricted activity is usually entirely satisfactory.

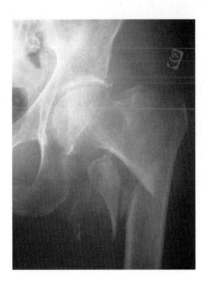

Figure 4.10 Radiograph of a left intertrochanteric neck of femur fracture.

Intertrochanteric fractures are extracapsular fractures in the plane between the greater and lesser trochanters. Closed reduction is usually possible using a traction table and the fracture can then undergo internal fixation using a cannulated hip screw. Union is usually rapid and pain relief after surgery excellent.

Subtrochanteric fractures occur through or distal to the lesser trochanter in essentially a transverse pattern. These fractures are unsuitable for management with plate fixation but lend themselves well to an intramedullary nail. Again rehabilitation tends to follow the same pattern as for intertrochanteric fractures.

Elderly patients cannot tolerate long periods of recumbency. Every effort should be made at the time of their admission to ensure that they are optimized for surgery. Delays arising from investigations not being carried out when the patient is admitted can have a great effect and a delay of even 24 hours to the patient receiving surgery can be problematic.

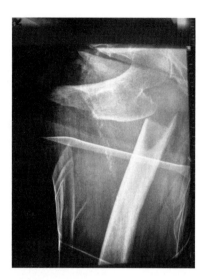

Figure 4.11 Radiograph of a subtrochanteric fracture.

OSCE Counselling cases

OSCE COUNSELLING CASE 4.3 – 'Doctor, I have a pin and plate in my leg. Do they need to be removed?'

Removal of metalwork was carried out routinely when operative surgical management of fractures first became an established part of treatment. However, it rapidly became apparent that this creates more problems than it solves.

Most orthopaedic trauma surgeons recommend the removal of metalwork in growing children. This prevents the metalwork becoming embedded in the growing bone, altering its mechanical properties and resulting in stress fractures, which present a very difficult surgical problem because of the presence of the embedded metalwork.

Removal of metalwork, however, is prone to problems with wound healing as a result of infection or haematoma formation, and also has the risk of peripheral nerve injury in the limb. This is particularly true of removal of forearm fracture plates.

Specific indications for removal of metalwork would include the following:

- Local pain caused by prominence of the metalwork under the skin
- Occasionally the removal of intramedullary nails in the lower limb long bone of high-class athletes because these can sometimes impair performance
- At a similar elite end of the scale, metalwork in the hand and wrist of accomplished musicians, because some authorities have reported that even the small changes caused by metalwork can interfere with performance (However, it should be borne in mind that this is true only for elite performers.)

Generally, metalwork in adults should stay in-situ provided that it is not responsible for any specific problems.

OSCE COUNSELLING CASE 4.4 – 'Doctor, with this open fracture of my tibia, am I going to lose my leg?'

Any fracture in the lower limb does have the potential to result in a loss of limb if its treatment or the fracture itself leads to complications; however, this is not normally the case.

Consider the likelihood of survival of someone sustaining an open tibial fracture as a result of the tsunami that struck Indonesia on Boxing Day 2004. By the time help arrived the casualty would almost certainly have died from either gangrene or tetanus. Such drastic infective complications are almost unheard of in developed countries with advanced medical care.

With appropriate management to convert the dirty traumatic wound into a clean surgical wound, and the unstable displaced fracture into a reduced stable fracture followed by reconstruction, after a short interval of 48 to 72 hours, of the soft tissue envelope, there is a considerable reduction in the risk of problems of non-union or infection and dramatic reduction in the risk of limb loss. Thus, although no guarantee can ever be given, the patient should be reassured that the chance of this happening is extremely low.

This question also presents an opportunity to challenge the patient about his or her concept of amputation. In the right circumstances amputation is an extremely good operation that can restore someone to independent mobility, free from pain, and to a nearly normal level of activity from a position where he or she had been severely disabled as a result of the injuries or their complications. It is most commonly required for patients whose fractures are associated with very severe soft tissue injuries, particularly those with nerve injuries, arterial injuries requiring repair and troublesome post-traumatic muscle contractures. Thus, amputation can be regarded as a method to improve a patient's quality of life from a severe injury.

REVISION PANEL

- In the case of a femoral shaft fracture, a Thomas splint can be applied in A&E which will provide instant pain relief.
- Radiographs of fractures should include the joint above and below the fracture site.
- Often, two views of a fracture such as anterior-posterior (AP) and lateral films will need to be obtained in order to assess the fracture pattern properly.
- Radiographs and full examination (including neurovascular status) of the injury site should be done before and after manipulation of the fracture and/or cast application.
- Open fractures must have prompt antibiotic administration, tetanus cover, be photographed, and taken to theatre as an emergency for wound debridement and washout in order to reduce the risk of infection.
- A comminuted fracture is where there are more than two bone components to the fracture. They commonly result from high-energy injuries.
- Blunting of sensation or pins and needles in an area around a fracture can indicate nerve damage or compression. It is particularly important to fully examine the patient and document your findings in these cases, *before and after* you manipulate the fracture.
- A patient who has tenderness in the anatomical snuffbox may have a scaphoid fracture. These fractures may not be visible on radiograph until a week after injury so it is important to follow up a patient in whom you suspect this diagnosis.
- A poly-trauma patient should be managed in accordance with ATLS guidelines, starting from first principles by managing airway, breathing and circulation as a priority.
- A large amount of blood can collect in the pelvis, which can lead to hypovolaemic shock. In a patient who is not maintaining his or her blood pressure despite fluid resuscitation with no obvious source of haemorrhage, consider bleeding into the pelvis and ensure a pelvic binder is on.
- In patients with a pelvic fracture, injury to the urinary tract, bowel, major blood vessels and nerves needs to be excluded due to the close proximity of these structures to the pelvic bones.
- Intracapsular fractures of the neck of femur and scaphoid are at risk of avascular necrosis due to the course of their blood supply which is often disrupted from the injury.
- When deciding on the management of a patient with a neck of femur fracture, treatment will be dependent on a patient's needs. The patient's mobility, if the patient is independent of activities of daily living, and past medical history will all be taken into account.
- Intracapsular neck of femur fractures are usually treated by total hip replacement or hemiarthroplasty. Extracapsular neck of femur fractures are often treated by cannulated hip screws or intramedullary devices dependent on fracture pattern.
- Implanted metalwork for fracture stabilization in children is often removed to prevent complications in later life. Implanted metalwork in adults is not routinely removed unless it is causing the patient pain due to the risks of performing such surgery.

BACK PROBLEMS

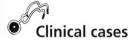

Clinical cases

For each of the clinical case scenarios given

Q1: What is the likely differential diagnosis?
Q2: What issues in the given history support the diagnosis?
Q3: What additional features in the history would you seek to support a particular diagnosis?
Q4: What clinical examination would you perform and why?
Q5: What investigations would be most helpful and why?
Q6: What treatment options are appropriate?

CASE 4.9 – **The teenager with thoracic back pain**

A 13-year-old girl has complained of increasing back pain in the lower thoracic/interscapular spine. This is aggravated by her schoolwork, in particular when she is doing homework. She is able to do games at school and this only moderately aggravates her symptoms.

CASE 4.10 – **The young adult with a trapped nerve**

A 32-year-old man had minor twinges of back pain over the course of the past week. Earlier today he was lifting his golf clubs out of the boot of his car when he experienced a searing pain and was unable to straighten up; he had severe pain radiating all the way from the back down to his right foot.

CASE 4.11 – **The pathological fracture**

A 72-year-old otherwise healthy woman had a minor fall when she slipped on some spilt milk on her tiled kitchen floor. She experienced very severe lower back pain and has been brought in by ambulance from home because she is unable to weight bear. She mentions that for the last couple of weeks she has had a strange woolly feeling in the right leg.

CASE 4.12 – **DIY gone wrong**

A 53-year-old man was attempting his own loft conversion and fell backwards through the loft hatch. He has severe lower back pain and has been brought in from home with spinal immobilization.

👥 OSCE Counselling cases

OSCE COUNSELLING CASE 4.5 – **'Doctor, I have terrible backache. The scan shows that I have a slipped disc. Don't I need an operation to take the slipped disc away?'**

Key concepts

THE SURGICAL SIEVE

- As mentioned before in the section 'The painful hip', the surgical sieve is helpful when approaching patients with back problems.
- Children and teenagers are most likely to have problems of developmental or rarely, but very importantly, malignant origin. Young adults tend to experience spinal problems associated with early degenerative change, and elderly people have problems caused by either osteoporosis or malignancy.
- Trauma, naturally, can affect any age group. Serious spinal injuries are very often seen after high-velocity or high-energy transfer road traffic accidents, or falls from heights by people attempting DIY.

Answers

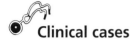
Clinical cases

CASE 4.9 – The teenager with thoracic back pain

A1: What is the likely differential diagnosis?

During the adolescent growth spurt aches and pains can come and go; however, if they are persistent they must be investigated because failure to recognize problems such as a slipped upper femoral epiphysis can be catastrophic.

A2: What issues in the given history support the diagnosis?

Thoracic back pain is either postural in origin or may result from Scheuermann's disease, an osteochondritic process affecting the midthoracic vertebrae, which is often asymptomatic and only discovered in later life as an incidental radiological finding. Another unlikely, but important, possibility is that of a malignant or infective process. Given that the patient in question is otherwise well and able to take part in activities, the most likely diagnosis is that of poor posture or Scheuermann's disease.

A3: What additional features in the history would you seek to support a particular diagnosis?

Malignancy affecting the thoracic spine is usually secondary to a previously known cancer; however, primary tumours do occur, originating in the bone marrow, or any of the musculoskeletal, vascular or neural elements of the spine. Rest pain and night pain support the diagnosis of infection or malignancy. The fact that posture (i.e. sitting at a desk and working) aggravates the symptoms strongly favours a purely mechanical origin. Other features indicating serious pathology are symptoms of nerve compression, altered sensation and altered power.

A4: What clinical examination would you perform and why?

The spine specifically should be examined with the patient standing, seated and lying prone. Neurological examination of the limbs would exclude any evidence of spinal or spinal nerve root involvement. Inspection of the spine will give a clear indication of any kyphotic changes that are commonly associated with Scheuermann's disease or lateral curvature of the spine – scoliosis – which may have remained undetected through the patient's early childhood. Postural scoliosis, which is habitual rather than a structural problem with the spine, will correct when the patient forward flexes to try to touch the floor. A true structural scoliosis will actually be accentuated by this manoeuvre. Careful palpation of the spine will elicit any areas of tenderness.

A5: What investigations would be most helpful and why?

Plain AP and lateral radiographs of the spine to include the whole spine should be taken if a structural scoliosis is defined. Then MRI would be indicated to further define any suggestion of bony destruction. Scheuermann's disease is recognized by simple anterior wedging of the thoracic vertebrae.

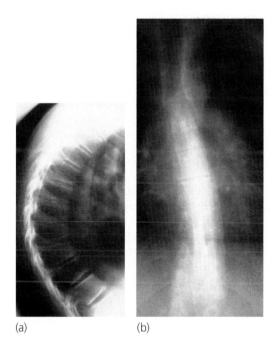

(a) (b)

Figure 4.12 Radiograph from a teenager with thoracic back pain: Scheuermann's disease.

A6: What treatment options are appropriate?

For management of Scheuermann's disease and thoracic pain of a purely postural origin, physiotherapy is all that is needed. The prognosis is excellent.

CASE 4.10 – **The young adult with a trapped nerve**

A1: What is the likely differential diagnosis?

The most likely differential diagnosis is that of a prolapsed intervertebral disc, which usually occurs at the level of L5/S1, trapping the S1 nerve root.

A2: What issues in the given history support the diagnosis?

A prolapsed intervertebral disc can occur against a long-standing history of mechanical back pain in young adults, with a simple event such as stooping to lift a comparatively light weight causing the degenerate disc to prolapse. This results in nerve root entrapment, inflammation and radicular pain as described.

A3: What additional features in the history would you seek to support a particular diagnosis?

Specific questions should be asked about previous episodes of lower back pain. In mechanical back pain, the lower back pain is a dominant symptom and such referred pain as the patient experiences is normally vague and referred into one or both thighs, usually anteriorly. The pain from a prolapsed disc resulting in nerve root entrapment is usually extreme. The resulting referred leg pain is worse than the back pain and may radiate all the way to the foot in the case of 'sciatica' or down to the knee in the front of thigh in the case of 'femoralgia'. Lower lumbar disc prolapses are much more common because the lower lumbar spine is subject to large stresses in ordinary everyday life. Femoralgia occurs as a result of a prolapsed disc higher in the lumbar spine and, although less common, is readily recognizable if it is sought.

A4: What clinical examination would you perform and why?

Neurological examination is mandatory. The patient may not be able to stand but should be encouraged to do so if he or she can. If possible the patient should be asked to walk on tiptoes. This is the most reliable way of assessing plantar flexion (S1 nerve root-innervated muscular strength). Careful inspection of the back will show the lumbar spine to have a loss of lordosis as a result of paraspinal muscle spasm and there will often be a scoliosis concave to the side in which the nerve root is entrapped, resulting from greater muscle spasm on that side.

Further clinical examination requires a thorough neurological examination of the patient's lower limbs plus saddle (urogenital/perianal) area, including digital rectal examination.

Tests for sciatic nerve root tension or femoral nerve root tension should be left until the end of the examination.

Power inhibition often occurs as a result of the extreme pain and so it is useful for the patient to be given a potent analgesic, before power testing is carried out.

In an L5 nerve root entrapment there may be weakness in great toe dorsiflexion and foot inversion. In an S1 nerve root entrapment there may be weakness in plantar flexion and foot eversion. The ankle jerk may be lost in either of the above cases. With femoralgia the quadriceps may be weak and there may be loss of the patellar tendon jerk. Sensory blunting is usually in a characteristic dermatomal distribution.

Examination of the perianal area is crucial. If the disc prolapse is central rather than lateral, cauda equina syndrome may result. In this case the patient will have no desire to void if nerve root entrapment affects those nerves mediating sensation to the bladder. Painless retention occurs and, unless surgical decompression is carried out urgently, incontinence and loss of sexual function will be permanent. Such patients usually have bilateral lower leg sciatic pain and bilateral perianal numbness with loss of anal tone. Careful clinical examination will often demonstrate the presence of a full bladder in a patient in whom there is no desire to void. Passage of a catheter is usually easy and pain free, with little sensation of catheter insertion experienced by the patient. A large volume of urine is usually drained.

Last, sciatic nerve root tension signs can be identified by the straight-leg raise. Care must be taken to do this gently and it is often a good idea to start with the pain-free leg, and to watch the patient's face. Lift the pain-free leg into the air gently, while encouraging the patient to relax. When he experiences pain enquire whether it is in the back or the ipsilateral or contralateral leg. Pain in the ipsilateral leg is a cross-over sign when examining the pain-free leg, suggesting a central disc prolapse. Keep the foot in its current position and then flex the knee. This should relieve leg pain. Note whether the pain is experienced solely in the back because this goes against sciatic nerve root tension.

Repeat the process with the contralateral leg. Bow-string signs and dorsiflexion of the foot to elicit pain again can also be performed after relieving pain by flexing the knee. However, the simple straight-leg raise test is normally enough to confirm or refute the diagnosis.

A5: What investigations would be most helpful and why?

A plain lateral radiograph of the lumbar spine is indicated to exclude any unexpected destructive malignant pathology. The gold standard investigation is MRI.

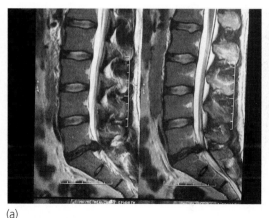 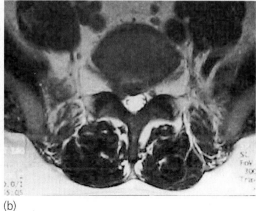

(a)   (b)

Figure 4.13 Young adult with a prolapsed intervertebral disc.

A6: What treatment options are appropriate?

In spite of the catastrophic nature of presentation most cases of sciatica will respond to analgesia supported by a muscle relaxant/antispasmodic and progressive physiotherapy. Long periods of bed rest should be avoided.

The patient should be encouraged to return to work as early as possible and to stop smoking. Interestingly, both of these are important features in long-term recovery.

In patients who fail these conservative measures a discectomy is indicated.

Cauda equina syndrome must be treated as an emergency. Urgent MRI should be performed with prompt spinal decompression by an appropriately skilled orthopaedic or neurosurgical spinal surgeon.

CASE 4.11 – **The pathological fracture**

A1: What is the likely differential diagnosis?

The differential diagnosis is restricted essentially to the diagnoses underlying pathological spinal fractures. The most common example would be an insufficiency fracture caused by osteoporosis.

Other origins of pathological weakness in the vertebrae include malignant deposits, which may be primary or secondary. A common primary deposit is myeloma. Secondary deposits usually originate in the breast, thyroid, lung, prostate or kidney.

A2: What issues in the given history support the diagnosis?

A history of previous insufficiency fractures would strongly support a diagnosis of an osteoporotic fracture. A history of a known malignancy would indicate the possibility of a tumour deposit.

In the given history the feeling of abnormal sensation in one lower limb hints at involvement of spinal nerve roots, which is not typical in osteoporotic fractures.

A3: What additional features in the history would you seek to support a particular diagnosis?

Specific questions should be asked about the past medical history to elicit the problems outlined above, plus general questions about the patient's overall health, well-being, weight loss etc.

A4: What clinical examination would you perform and why?

Clinical examination should be performed with the patient lying supine and carrying out the spinal immobilization precautions for the injured area. It must be presumed, in the presence of a fall, a history suggestive of a fracture and abnormal neurological symptoms, that the spinal injury is potentially unstable. Further movement without appropriate care could easily result in worsening neurological damage.

Otherwise neurological examination should be carried out exactly as for Case 4.10.

A5: What investigations would be most helpful and why?

Plain radiographs are essential, and may demonstrate a simple wedge compression consistent with an osteoporotic insufficiency fracture. In the history presented, it is quite possible that the AP view of the lumbar spine would demonstrate loss of the pedicle at the level of the fracture – a radiological finding suggestive of malignant destruction.

Further investigations should include FBC, ESR, biochemistry screen including liver function tests, CRP, urine for Bence Jones proteins and protein electrophoresis of the serum.

Magnetic resonance imaging is mandatory to define the extent of any soft tissue mass associated with a pathological fracture and to assist in planning of surgery for decompression of such a mass and stabilization of the spine to allow for mobilization of the patient.

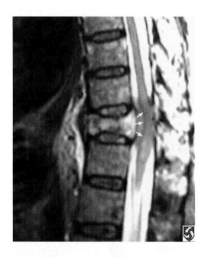

Figure 4.14 Radiograph showing a pathological spinal fracture.

A6: What treatment options are appropriate?

If the woman's fracture is entirely attributable to osteoporotic change, she simply needs to be given analgesia and gently and progressively mobilized thereafter. Care should be taken to ensure that she has appropriate treatment for her osteoporosis to help reduce the risks of further fractures.

In the case of spinal cord or spinal nerve root compression with an associated fracture caused by a malignant deposit, surgical decompression after pre-operative treatment with steroids to reduce associated tumour-related swelling would have a reasonable chance of restoring lower limb function in this woman. The more severe the pre-operative nerve impairment, the less the chance of complete resolution of symptoms with spinal decompression and operative stabilization of the spine – hence the importance of careful handling of the patient pre-operatively.

CASE 4.12 – **DIY gone wrong**

A1: What is the likely differential diagnosis?

The most likely differential diagnosis is a burst fracture – an unstable fracture of one of the lumbar vertebrae; less likely is a stable wedge compression fracture.

A2: What issues in the given history support the diagnosis?

It is impossible from the history to determine whether the fracture sustained is stable or unstable unless there is neurological injury. Neurological injury is a sign that the associated fracture is unstable.

A3: What additional features in the history would you seek to support a particular diagnosis?

Not applicable

A4: What clinical examination would you perform and why?

Full spinal precautions must be taken, including immobilization of the cervical spine.

The patient should have a thorough neurological examination in the supine position, paying particular attention to loss of sensation, reflexes and power in the lower limbs, and the urogenital triangle as described above.

In addition, specific examination of the feet, ankles, knees and hips should be carried out because in a fall from a height, typical associated injuries include fractures of the calcaneum, distal articular surface of the tibia (plafond), tibial plateau, femoral condyles, hips and pelvis.

A5: What investigations would be most helpful and why?

Plain radiographs will help confirm the level of the spinal fracture and may give important information as to whether or not, in the patient who is neurologically intact, the fracture is stable.

It is important to understand that a fracture may be completely unstable but the patient neurologically completely normal.

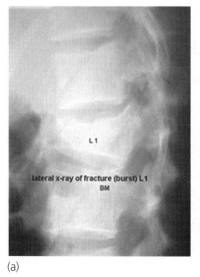
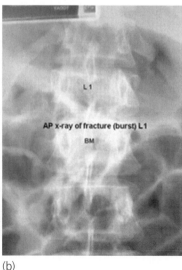

(a)   (b)

Figure 4.15 Radiographs showing a fracture of L1 (a) lateral view (b) AP view.

Features suggesting instability include loss of the anterior vertebral body height: greater than 30 per cent of the posterior vertebral body height suggests posterior element injuries. Again this hints at the potential for unstable motion of this injured spinal segment.

On the AP radiograph, wedging in the lateral direction suggests a rotational rather than a true wedge compression mechanism, further indicating instability. Clear-cut signs of instability on the plain radiographs are those of a retropulsed fragment encroaching on the spinal canal and loss of posterior vertebral height; both of these features are visible on the lateral view. On the AP view, the signs are widening of the distance between the pedicles in comparison to the vertebrae above and below.

Computed tomography will define the precise architecture of the bones at this level and facilitate planning of spinal surgery if this is deemed necessary.

Further radiographs should be carried out of the feet, tibial plateaux, hips, pelvis and so on if areas of tenderness or deformity have been identified.

A6: What treatment options are appropriate?

Full spinal immobilization should be continued until the spine either is recognized as being stable or becomes stable through healing or surgical intervention.

OSCE Counselling case

OSCE COUNSELLING CASE 4.5 – **'Doctor, I have terrible backache. The scan shows that I have a slipped disc. Don't I need an operation to take the slipped disc away?'**

Surgery for prolapsed discs does not cure back pain. The indication for surgery to remove a prolapsed disc, or rather that portion of the disc that has prolapsed, is chronic back pain that fails to settle with appropriate conservative measures including a very committed, specific physiotherapy programme.

In such cases discectomy is by and large successful in relieving leg pain but has little or no impact on back pain. Long-term follow-up studies of patients undergoing surgical versus non-surgical management for sciatica in relation to prolapsed lumbar discs show that there is no overall difference in outcome.

There are specific risks associated with discectomy and these include nerve root injury at the time of surgery, chronic fibrosis as a consequence of surgical intervention and more immediate problems such as epidural haematoma, which can lead to paraplegia, although this is exceedingly rare.

A degenerate disc that leads to a disabled motion segment in the spine is occasionally a source of back pain, which can be managed with spinal fusion. The risks of spinal fusion surgery are similar to, but greater than, those of simple discectomy, and hence every effort should be made to optimize patients' conditions through non-surgical means; patients should be well informed about the risks of any surgery that they consider.

REVISION PANEL

- Scheuermann's disease is an osteochondritic process that can cause back pain in some individuals and no symptoms in others. Kyphotic changes of the spine will often be present and on radiograph simple anterior wedging of the thoracic vertebrae will be seen.
- A prolapsed intervertebral disc often occurs in a patient who has had a long-standing history of mechanical back pain. Symptoms will be dependent on the severity of the prolapse and what nerve root(s) are compressed. A full neurological examination is mandatory.
- Cauda equina syndrome must be treated as an emergency with urgent examination, imaging, and if necessary, decompression surgery to avoid long-term disability.
- Osteoporotic insufficiency fractures are usually seen as wedge compression fractures on radiograph.
- Signs of an unstable vertebral fracture on radiograph include wedging in the lateral direction, a retropulsed fragment encroaching on the spinal canal, loss of posterior vertebral height, and widening of the distance between the pedicles in comparison to the vertebrae above and below.

ACKNOWLEDGEMENT

The contribution of Ian Pallister to this chapter in the first edition is gratefully acknowledged.

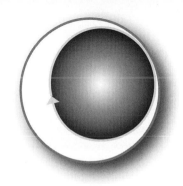

5 Urology

Suresh Ganta

PROSTATE CANCER AND PSA

INCONTINENCE

NEUROPATHIC BLADDER

UPPER TRACT OBSTRUCTION AND RENAL MASS

SCROTAL PAIN, TESTICULAR LUMPS

ERECTILE DYSFUNCTION/INFERTILITY

HAEMATURIA

Questions

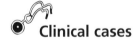 **Clinical cases**

For each of the clinical case scenarios given

> **Q1:** What is the likely differential diagnosis?
> **Q2:** What issues in the given history support/refute a particular diagnosis?
> **Q3:** What additional features would you seek to support a particular diagnosis?
> **Q4:** What clinical examination would you perform and why?
> **Q5:** What investigations would be most helpful and why?
> **Q6:** What treatment options are appropriate?

CASE 5.1 – 'I can see blood in my urine'

A 65-year-old man presents to his general practitioner (GP) with painless total haematuria with some clots. He has no associated urinary symptoms. He has been a moderate smoker for the last 40 years and worked in a chemical factory for 25 years. He has noticed a half-stone weight loss (about 3 kg) over the last 4 months.

CASE 5.2 – 'I have to go quite frequently and also have blood in my urine'

A 35-year-old woman presents with dysuria and hourly urinary frequency. She has significant urgency and terminal haematuria. She has suprapubic discomfort and a feeling of incomplete emptying of her bladder. She has also had flu-like symptoms over the last 2 days. She has two children and is a smoker.

CASE 5.3 – 'There is blood on testing my urine'

A 37-year-old businessman has an insurance medical health check and is found to have blood in his urine with a dipstick test. He is completely asymptomatic. He does not smoke and has had no urinary symptoms.

👫 OSCE Counselling case

OSCE COUNSELLING CASE 5.1 – 'How do I prevent recurrent urine infections?'

A 45-year-old woman presents with recurrent urinary infections. She has had three vaginal deliveries and required a forceps delivery for the last child who is now aged 18 years. She has noticed some stress leakage of urine and has a mild vaginal prolapse.

Key concepts

HAEMATURIA

This is the presence of blood in the urine and is confirmed by the presence of >10 to 20 red blood cells (RBCs)/mL in the urine. Macroscopic (frank, visible) haematuria is more serious because it is more often associated with pathology than microscopic haematuria. It may be either associated with symptoms of bladder irritability and pain, or painless. Painless haematuria may be the only symptom of an underlying cancer. Surprisingly, less than 50 per cent of patients presenting with macroscopic haematuria are found to have a serious underlying disease.

Types of haematuria

- Initial haematuria usually arises from the urethra. It occurs least commonly and is usually secondary to inflammation.
- Total haematuria is most common and indicates bleeding from either the bladder or upper tracts.
- Terminal haematuria occurs at the end of micturition and usually from bladder neck or prostate and occurs when the bladder neck contracts and squeezes all residual urine.

BLADDER CANCER

This commonly presents with painless macroscopic haematuria (90 per cent). In 10 per cent of cases presenting with bladder cancer, microscopic haematuria is the only presenting symptom. Transitional cell carcinoma is the most common type of bladder cancer in Europe and the United States.

Bladder tumours are graded according to cytological and nuclear features into well differentiated (G1), intermediately differentiated (G2) and poorly differentiated (G3).

Tumours are staged according to the depth of invasion into the muscle wall:

- pTa: non-invasive papillary carcinoma confined to the lamina propria
- pT1: tumour invades the subepithelial connective tissue known as the lamina propria
- pT2: tumour invades muscle (called the detrusor muscle)
- pT3: tumour invades perivesical tissue
- pT4: tumour invades prostate, uterus, vagina or pelvic or abdominal wall.

Treatment depends on the stage and grade of the tumour as well as the general condition of the patient. Non-invasive (pTa, pTis, pT1) tumours are mainly managed by endoscopic resection and intravesical treatment with chemotherapy or immunotherapy. The main options for muscle invasive tumours (pT2 and above) are managed by surgery to remove the bladder or radiotherapy to the bladder with or without chemotherapy.

Answers

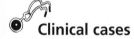

Clinical cases

CASE 5.1 – 'I can see blood in my urine'

A1: What is the likely differential diagnosis?

- Bladder cancer
- Bleeding from the prostate
- Renal carcinoma
- Bladder stone
- Cystitis

A2: What issues in the given history support/refute a particular diagnosis?

Frank haematuria has a 20 per cent probability of detecting an underlying urological malignancy. Ninety per cent of bladder cancers present with haematuria. Pain may be absent with malignancy and is usually associated with an inflammatory process causing haematuria. Smoking and occupational exposure to chemicals such as aromatic amines in the leather/textile/rubber/paint industry are known risk factors for bladder cancer. Renal tumours are more often discovered incidentally by imaging of the abdomen for other reasons. The typical triad of symptoms with loin pain, mass and haematuria are only present in 11 per cent of patients with renal tumours.

A3: What additional features would you seek to support a particular diagnosis?

The duration and severity of bleeding would determine the need to resuscitate. The timing of haematuria often indicates the site of origin (e.g. initial, total and terminal haematuria). Clots in the urine often indicate severity and may also cause clot retention of urine. The shape of clots (e.g. vermicular [worm like]) often associated with pain may be related to upper ureteric (from ureter). The most common cause of gross haematuria in the older population is bladder cancer.

A4: What clinical examination would you perform and why?

Clinical examination is performed to determine blood loss (e.g. pallor), plus complete physical examination to identify abdominal masses and digital rectal examination (DRE) to examine the prostate.

A5: What investigations would be most helpful and why?

- Urine microscopy: to rule out infection, glomerular haematuria (from renal glomerulus) is associated with dysmorphic (abnormal shapes of red blood cells) red cell casts. Crystals in urine may suggest stone disease. Parasites and ova may be noted in the urine (schistosomiasis).
- Urine cytology: There is a high specificity (96 per cent) to identify transitional cell cancer of the urinary tract but low overall sensitivity (<75 per cent). It is particularly useful in cases of carcinoma in situ of the bladder and for high-grade tumours.
- NMP-22 relies on identifying nuclear matrix protein in urine as a tumour marker in urine. UroVysion® is a urinary marker that uses fluorescence in situ hybridization (FISH) to identify certain chromosomal foci to identify tumour cells and has high specificity (75 per cent) and sensitivity (98 per cent).
- Intravenous urogram (IVU)/CT urography: identifies anatomy and function of the upper tracts. Contrast is injected into the vein and this is filtered in the kidney into the collecting system of

the urinary tract. Then CT scans of the abdomen and pelvis may identify anatomy and delay in accumulation in the collecting system.
- Ultrasonography: identifies abnormality of renal parenchyma.
- Cystoscopy: 'gold standard' for assessment of the bladder – flexible cystoscopy under local anaesthetic or a rigid cystoscopy under general anaesthetic. This identifies the site of bleeding and whether biopsy/resection is possible.

A6: What treatment options are appropriate?

Bladder tumours are diagnosed and staged after trans-urethral resection of the bladder tumour (TURBT) and complete removal. The diagnosis of the bladder tumour often describes the cell type (e.g. transitional cell type, 90 per cent; adenocarcinoma, 2 per cent; squamous cell type, 5 per cent), depth of invasion, and grade of the cancer. Further imaging (e.g. computed tomography [CT]) may be appropriate in certain cases with larger tumours, to assess the extent of invasion into the bladder muscle wall and the distant spread.

Superficial bladder tumours (80 per cent, non-muscle invasive) are prone to recurrence after endoscopic treatment and ablation of the tumour. This is due to a urothelial field change by a combination of genetic factors and external risk factors. The rate of developing further recurrences depends on the size of the largest tumour, number of tumours, T category, grade of tumour at diagnosis, and whether a recurrence was noted at 3 months after the primary resection.

A bladder tumour is more likely to progress both in terms of stage progression (Ta to T1/T1 to T2) and grade progression (G1 to G2/G2 to G3). Progression affects overall and disease-specific survival.

MANAGEMENT

Superficial bladder cancer (Tis, Ta, T1)

- Small, solitary, low-grade mucosal diploid tumours (Ta)
  - Low risk or recurrence
  - TURBT followed by a single dose of intravesical chemotherapy
  - Surveillance for recurrence by cystoscopy
- Multifocal, high-grade aneuploid tumours (Tis or T1)
  - TURBT followed by a single dose of intravesical chemotherapy
  - Intravesical immunotherapy/chemotherapy (single post-operative dose or every week for 6 weeks):
    - Bacille Calmette–Guérin (BCG) for grade 3 superficial bladder cancer G3pTa/pT1 or Tis (carcinoma in situ)
    - Intravesical course of chemotherapy (e.g. mitomycin)

Invasive bladder cancer (T1–T4)

- Neo-adjuvant chemotherapy followed by radical cystectomy with pelvic lymphadenectomy and urinary diversion
- Neo-adjuvant chemotherapy followed by external beam bladder irradiation
- Systemic chemotherapy using M-VAC (methotrexate/vinblastine sulfate/doxorubicin [adriamycin]/cis-platinum)

Metastatic bladder cancer

- Chemotherapy
  - M-VAC/paclitaxel-based chemotherapy
  - Gemcitabine/cis-platinum

Untreated metastatic bladder cancer has a 2-year survival rate of <5 per cent.

CASE 5.2 – 'I have to go quite frequently and also have blood in my urine'

A1: What is the likely differential diagnosis?
- Urinary tract infection (UTI)
- Carcinoma in situ of the bladder
- Interstitial cystitis
- Bladder stones or lower ureteric stone

A2: What issues in the given history support/refute a particular diagnosis?
- Dysuria and frequency
- Suprapubic pain or discomfort, common to patients with cystitis
- Feeling an incomplete emptying of bladder, with flu-like symptoms

A3: What additional features would you seek to support a particular diagnosis?
Recurrent infections often have an underlying predisposing cause. They are common in sexually active women but also occur in older postmenopausal women prone to constipation and immobility. Bladder outflow obstruction typically presents with a reduced urine flow, frequency and incomplete bladder emptying, with a high post-micturition residual volume. A history of diabetes, uterine prolapse, recent urethral instrumentation, indwelling long-term urethral catheters or stents and urinary stone disease is relevant.

Ureteric reflux of urine is another cause of re-infection and may be associated with an ascending infection (pyelonephritis), which typically presents with loin pain, fever and being systemically unwell.

A4: What clinical examination would you perform and why?
- General examination to assess sepsis and dehydration
- Abdominal examination for masses or palpable bladder
- Vaginal examination for prolapse (in men a rectal examination to assess the prostate)

A5: What investigations would be most helpful and why?
- Dipstick:
  - Leukocyte esterase test: detects pus cells in the urine
  - Nitrate reductase test: detects bacteria that reduce nitrate to nitrite (specificity of >90 per cent but sensitivity is variable at 35 to 80 per cent)
- Urine microscopy and culture: a colony count of 100 000/cc is used to define infection and to identify organism and antimicrobial sensitivity. It is important to note that significant infection may exist even with a colony count of 1000/cc and a midstream urine specimen free of contamination is essential to aid diagnosis.
- Urine cytology: this is particularly useful in the presence of storage lower urinary tract symptoms in the context of recurrent UTIs to rule out transitional cell carcinoma (TCC) of the urinary bladder.
- Plain radiograph of the abdomen: this identifies renal tract calcification.
- Ultrasonography of renal tract: this assesses renal cortex thickness and scarring (common after recurrent ascending infections) and measures post-micturition residual in the bladder.
- Contrast CT urography or intravenous urogram (IVU): this defines the anatomy of renal tract and stone disease.
- Cystoscopy: this is performed if persistent haematuria is present or there are significant storage lower urinary tract symptoms.

● Micturating cystourethrogram: this is indicated only if renal scarring is noted and clinical features suggest ureteric reflux.

A6: What treatment options are appropriate?

It is important to classify UTIs into uncomplicated, complicated or recurrent ones. An uncomplicated UTI is one that occurs in a healthy woman with a structurally and functionally normal urinary tract. This is often treated empirically with a short course of broad-spectrum antibiotics followed by appropriate treatment based on urine cultures, which often take 2 to 3 days. Further investigations are needed if there are three episodes of cystitis in women and a single episode of infection in men.

A complicated urine infection is considered if factors like male gender, childhood UTI, pregnancy, immunocompromised, elderly and indwelling foreign body (e.g. catheter) or abnormal urinary tract are present. A recurrent infection is often due to resistant organisms and requires a modified approach, often with advice from a microbiologist.

Treat predisposing causes such as obstruction (urethral dilatation if the urethra is stenosed), correction of uncontrolled diabetes, treatment of stone disease and prolapse. Bacterial adherence to the urothelium or vaginal epithelium is an essential step in initiation of UTI. This is determined by several bacterial adhesins (e.g. pili on surface of bacteria) that may be on the surface of urinary pathogenic *Escherichia coli* that bind to the epithelial cells. The adhesive characteristics of the epithelial cells of women susceptible to infections and pathogenic bacteria are associated with increased risk of infection. Bladder wall epithelium permeability and adherence is reduced by exogenous glycosaminoglycans (GAG) (e.g. hyaluronic acid).

CASE 5.3 – 'There is blood on testing my urine'

A1: What is the likely differential diagnosis?

Causes of asymptomatic microscopic haematuria by incidence are as follows:

● Benign essential haematuria (37 per cent)
● Benign prostatic hyperplasia (BPH) (24 per cent)
● UTI (27 per cent)
● Urinary stone disease (6 per cent)
● Bladder tumour (2 per cent)
● Renal cyst (1.5 per cent)
● Renal tumour (0.5 per cent)

A2: What issues in the given history support/refute a particular diagnosis?

A nephrological cause for microscopic haematuria is common in those aged under 40 years and may be associated with hypertension and proteinuria.

A3: What additional features would you seek to support a particular diagnosis?

● Benign causes:
  ● UTI
  ● Trauma, vigorous exercise-induced haematuria, menstruation and sexual activity
● Nephrological cause:
  ● Is there young-onset hypertension?
  ● Is there proteinuria?
  ● Renal insufficiency
● Red cell casts or dysmorphic red cells in urine

Risk factors for significant disease with microscopic haematuria:

- Smoking
- Occupational exposure to chemicals or dyes (benzenes or aromatic amines)
- History of urological disease or storage lower urinary tract symptoms (LUTS) and UTI
- Analgesic abuse
- History of pelvic irradiation

A4: What clinical examination would you perform and why?

Examine for abdominal masses and any pelvic masses, including assessment of prostate.

A5: What investigations would be most helpful and why?

- Urine microscopy: rules out infection
- Urine phase contrast microscopy: for dysmorphic erythrocytes indicating glomerular source of bleeding
- Urine cytology: identifies transitional cell carcinoma
- CT urography/IVU or ultrasonography: for assessing the anatomy of the renal tract and collecting system
- Renal biopsy: rarely indicated and usually supervised by a nephrologist
- Cystoscopy: the 'gold standard' investigation for the bladder

A6: What treatment options are appropriate?

The incidence of underlying urological malignancy in those presenting with microscopic haematuria is 5 to 7 per cent; it is therefore important to investigate all patients with microscopic haematuria. The risk of underlying malignancy increases with age, and those over 55 years with microscopic haematuria are referred as urgent 2-week referrals.

A patient with asymptomatic microscopic haematuria, proteinuria and hypertension who is aged under 40 years is likely to have a glomerular cause for the microscopic haematuria. Immunoglobulin IgA nephropathy is the most common cause found on renal biopsy when no urological cause is noted.

Glomerular causes:

- Age <50 years
  - IgA nephropathy
  - Thin basement membrane disease
  - Alport's disease (hereditary nephritis)
  - Mild focal glomerulonephritis (GN)
- Age >50 years
  - IgA nephropathy
  - Alport's disease (hereditary nephritis)
  - Mild focal GN

Referral to a nephrologist is recommended if risk factors for underlying nephrological cause are present.

Investigation of asymptomatic microscopic haematuria may also reveal an underlying urological pathology such as urinary stone disease, infections, BPH or urological cancer that is treated appropriately.

‍ OSCE Counselling case

OSCE COUNSELLING CASE 5.1 – 'How do I prevent recurrent urinary infections?'

Re-infection with the same strain of the organism is more common than persistence of the urinary pathogen. Colonic or perineal flora are the reservoir for these re-infecting strains. A relapse within 7 days of treatment usually indicates failure to eradicate the infection. In contrast, if bacteriuria is absent 14 days after infection and followed by a recurrence of infection, this is likely to be a re-infection. It is therefore essential to treat every infection with the appropriate antibiotic for an adequate length of time to prevent relapse.

General measures to prevent infections include adequate fluid intake, appropriate frequent voiding and postcoital micturition. It is good to achieve a short voiding interval and high flow rate, drinking large amounts of fluid to dilute the bacteria.

Regular intake of cranberry juice has been shown to be helpful in reducing recurrent infections.

Although not proven, excessive scrubbing and cleaning may damage genital skin and vaginal mucous membranes by excessive douching and reduce the normal barrier to infection.

Wiping the anus from front to back after passing stools should be encouraged as general hygiene principles.

Investigation and treatment should consider the predisposing factors such as stones, urethral diverticulum and diabetes.

REVISION PANEL

- Bladder cancer is one of the most common causes of visible painless haematuria.
- Transitional cell cancer is the most common form of bladder cancer with squamous and adenocarcinoma.
- Superficial or non-muscle invasive bladder cancer is managed by endoscopic resection followed by intravesical chemotherapy. Recurrences are managed by endoscopic surveillance and by intravesical chemotherapy.
- Muscle invasive bladder cancer is managed by radical treatment with either radical cystectomy or radical radiotherapy to the bladder.
- Uncomplicated UTI is often in healthy women with a structurally and functionally normal urinary tract. It is often treated empirically with a short course of antibiotics from 1 to 3 days.
- Complicated UTI is often in men, children and pregnant women or is associated with abnormal urinary tract, immunocompromised or with indwelling foreign bodies. This often requires a longer course of antibiotics.
- Recurrent UTIs are associated with a range of causes like atrophic vaginitis, abnormal urinary tract or poor bladder emptying. Bacterial adherence is associated with increased virulence and altering the adhesins.
- Microscopic haematuria in those <40 years of age is usually due to nephrological causes.
- Microscopic haematuria may be due to underlying malignancy and the risk increases with age and hence in >55 years of age is referred as a 2-week referral.
- Microscopic haematuria is investigated with lower tract cystoscopy and upper tract imaging.

STONE DISEASE

Questions

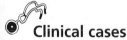
Clinical cases

For each of the clinical case scenarios given

Q1: What is the likely differential diagnosis?
Q2: What issues in the given history support/refute a particular diagnosis?
Q3: What additional features would you seek to support a particular diagnosis?
Q4: What clinical examination would you perform and why?
Q5: What investigations would be most helpful and why?
Q6: What treatment options are appropriate?

CASE 5.4 – 'I have pain in my loin'

A 45-year-old woman presents to her GP with significant loin pain associated with nausea and vomiting. She has had a similar episode before and has required an operation to remove a stone in her ureter.

CASE 5.5 – 'I have recurrent infection and a dull ache in my loin'

A 35-year-old woman presents with dysuria and passing stones/debris in her urine. She also has a dull loin ache. She has had recurrent UTIs that her GP has been treating with antibiotics for the last 2 years. She has two children and is a smoker.

CASE 5.6 – 'I have a fever and quite severe pain in my loin'

A 37-year-old businessman had quite severe pain in his loin with a high temperature and was feeling unwell.

👥 OSCE Counselling cases

OSCE COUNSELLING CASE 5.2 – 'How do I prevent recurrent stone formation?'

A 45-year-old woman presents with a 4-year history of recurrent urine infections. She has had two normal deliveries and has a normal menstrual cycle. Clinical examination and investigations are unremarkable.

Q1: What general measures would you recommend to reduce urine infections?

OSCE COUNSELLING CASE 5.3 – 'How do I counsel for extracorporeal shock wave lithotripsy (ESWL)?'

Key concepts

PRESENTATION

- Renal pain is usually felt in the loin, sometimes spreading to the umbilicus and testis.
- Obstruction of the lower ureter may lead to bladder irritability or pain in the scrotum, penile tip or labia majora. Stones can also cause a recurrent painful desire to micturate, with only a little urine passed each time (strangury).

PREDISPOSING FACTORS FOR STONE FORMATION

- Low urine volume can contribute to stone formation.
- Metabolic disorders of calcium: absorptive hypercalciuria is the most common abnormality detected in patients with calcium oxalate stones and is present in about 60 per cent of such patients. It is caused by an altered intestinal response to vitamin D, leading to increased absorption of calcium and hypercalcaemia, and decreased parathyroid hormone (PTH) secretion.
- Elevated urinary excretion/concentration of oxalate, calcium or uric acid; decreased excretion of inhibitors of stone growth; increase in urinary pH all contribute to stone formation.

BASIC ADVICE AND TREATMENT FOR RECURRENT STONE FORMERS

The most important risk factor is urine volume: if the volume is doubled, the risk of forming further stones is reduced by a factor of four.

CRYSTALLINE COMPOSITION OF RENAL CALCULI

- Calcium oxalate (40 per cent)
- Calcium phosphate (15 per cent)
- Mixed oxalate/phosphate (20 per cent)
- Struvite (15 per cent)
- Uric acid (10 per cent)
- Miscellaneous stones 15 per cent (cystine, rare metabolites, drugs etc.)

Analysis of a stone to determine composition can be useful in the management of patients with renal stones.

Answers

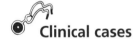 **Clinical cases**

CASE 5.4 – 'I have pain in my loin'

A1: What is the likely differential diagnosis?

- Ureteric colic
- Acute appendicitis
- Diverticulitis
- Ruptured aortic aneurysm
- Salpingitis
- Pyelonephritis

A2: What issues in the given history support/refute a particular diagnosis?

- History is consistent with ureteric colic (e.g. radiating loin to groin pain). Pain is often continuous. Pain from obstruction to upper or mid ureteric stone may cause pain on the right side in keeping with right iliac fossa pain mimicking acute appendicitis. Pain from mid-ureteric obstruction on the left side causes pain in the left iliac fossa mimicking acute diverticulitis. Pain from lower ureteric obstruction may cause pain to the tip of the penis or labia and often may have frequency and urgency.
- Haematuria on urinalysis and persistent pain are recorded.

A3: What additional features would you seek to support a particular diagnosis?

History suggestive of a ureteric colic may be associated with fever in pyelonephritis. The presence of obstruction with infection in a renal unit leads to severe systemic sepsis and is particularly important to rule out the presence of hydronephrosis. The presence of hydronephrosis may suggest obstruction and drainage of the renal unit with either a nephrostomy or insertion of a ureteric stent may be required. Ureteric obstruction leads to nephron loss in the affected renal unit. The presence of infection accelerates the nephron loss extremely rapidly and drainage of the renal unit is essential to reduce nephron loss.

Criteria for admission:

- Pain not adequately controlled
- Temperature >37.5°C and signs of sepsis/obstructed kidney/unstable patient
- Unable to tolerate diet and fluids
- Deranged urea and electrolytes (U&Es) and raised white blood cell count (WCC)

A4: What clinical examination would you perform and why?

A ruptured abdominal aortic aneurysm may cause loin pain and may mimic a ureteric colic particularly in older patients and hence a high index of suspicion needs to be maintained. Therefore, an abdominal examination for pulsatile mass or aneurysm is essential. Identification of bruising in the loin is associated with retroperitoneal bleeding (e.g. ruptured aortic aneurysm). Clinical examination reveals renal tenderness and renal mass. Pain, renal mass and haematuria may be associated with a renal tumour.

A5: What investigations would be most helpful and why?

- Urine microscopy is used to rule out infection.

- IVU shows 90 per cent of stones which are radio-opaque. It is useful to assess the anatomy and function of the urinary tract and also identify the size of stone and the degree and level of obstruction.
- Computed tomography (helical/spiral CT) is the current 'gold standard' for imaging abdominal pain and can identify ureteric calculi and other causes of abdominal pain. It has a sensitivity and specificity of 96 per cent and 100 per cent, respectively.

A6: What treatment options are appropriate?

Symptomatic treatment, analgesia, antibiotics, drainage of kidney using either a percutaneous nephrostomy or ureteric JJ stent insertion. Prompt drainage of the kidney (e.g. percutaneous nephrostomy/JJ stent insertion) is indicated in a patient with an obstructed, infected upper urinary tract, impending renal deterioration, intractable pain or vomiting, anuria or high-grade obstruction of a solitary or transplanted kidney.

CASE 5.5 – 'I have recurrent infection and a dull ache in my loin'

A1: What is the likely differential diagnosis?
- Pelviureteric junction (PUJ) obstruction
- Urinary stone disease
- Ureteric reflux disease
- Xanthogranulomatous pyelonephritis (XGPN)
- Renal tract tuberculosis (TB)

A2: What issues in the given history support/refute a particular diagnosis?

Recurrent UTIs, fever, passing grit and stones

A3: What additional features would you seek to support a particular diagnosis?

A history of loin pain after increased fluid intake and alcohol would suggest obstruction of the PUJ.

Xanthogranulomatous pyelonephritis represents an unusual suppurative granulomatous reaction to chronic infection, often in the presence of chronic obstruction from a calculus, stricture or tumour, and may present with symptoms of long-standing inflammation and loin pain in patients with urinary stone disease. Both CT and ultrasonography show areas of pus and necrotic debris within the kidney.

Renal tract TB, although uncommon in the United Kingdom, should be considered. Pulmonary TB precedes the development of genitourinary TB.

A4: What clinical examination would you perform and why?

Abdominal examination should be performed to rule out renal mass. Loin bruising or swelling may suggest retroperitoneal collection of blood or pus. Pus may tract along the psoas major and present as a collection in the groin.

A5: What investigations would be most helpful and why?
- Radiograph of the abdomen: identifies renal tract calcifications
- Ultrasonography: hydronephrosis and dilatation of renal pelvis
- IVU: function and anatomy of the renal tract
- CT urography: will identify renal anatomy
- Technetium-99m-labelled mercaptoacetyl triglycine (MAG-3): identifies the presence of underlying obstruction to the kidney and split function of the kidney

A6: What treatment options are appropriate?

Staghorn calculi require a multimodal approach to their treatment and often need more than one procedure to ensure complete removal, which is necessary because residual stone fragments quite rapidly form a nidus for further stone formation.

Struvite stones are invariably associated with urinary infections – specifically, the presence of urease-producing bacteria, including Ureaplasma urealyticum and Proteus spp. (most common). These lead to the hydrolysis of urea into ammonium and hydroxyl ions, resulting in an alkaline urine. The resultant increase in ammonium and phosphate concentrations combined with the alkaline urine (pH > 7.2) are necessary for struvite and carbonate apatite crystallization.

Treatment includes antimicrobials to reduce infection, and urinary acidifying agents to reduce stone formation.

A combination of extracorporeal shock wave lithotripsy (ESWL) and percutaneous nephrolithotomy (PCNL) is used to treat staghorn calculi.

Chemolytic therapy may be used either as a local irrigation via a nephrostomy or as oral agents. The latter have a role in patients who are not candidates for surgical removal of calculi and are also used as adjunctive therapy to dissolve residual apatite or struvite calculi and fragments after surgery, or to achieve partial dissolution of renal calculi to facilitate surgical removal.

Rarely open surgical treatment becomes necessary for the removal of large, complex renal calculi – either anatrophic nephrolithotomy (bivalving the kidney on the lateral aspect) or pyelolithotomy (opening the renal pelvis).

CASE 5.6 – 'I have a fever and quite severe pain in my loin'

A1: What is the likely differential diagnosis?

Upper UTI is likely: pyelonephritis is commonly associated with loin pain, fever and rigors. High-grade obstruction with infection in an obstructed renal system is commonly associated with severe pain and rapid septicaemia. In this case the patient will be very sick with hypotension, poor peripheral perfusion and circulatory collapse.

A2: What issues in the given history support/refute a particular diagnosis?

Stone disease and being unwell with fever would suggest infection and possible obstruction of the ureter. The presence of hydronephrosis often signifies obstruction (although dilatation of the collecting system may not always be synonymous with obstruction).

A3: What additional features would you seek to support a particular diagnosis?

History of diabetes or immunosuppression is important as a predisposing factor.

Infection with a gas-forming organism is not uncommon in patients with diabetes – 'emphysematous pyelonephritis'. This has a high mortality rate. It is diagnosed radiologically by the presence of gas in the parenchyma or collecting system and is managed surgically.

A4: What clinical examination would you perform and why?

The patient is usually very ill with fever, chills, flank pain and tenderness, and severe sepsis-related circulatory collapse.

Infected hydronephrosis is bacterial infection in a hydronephrotic kidney and pyonephrosis is suppurative destruction of parenchyma of kidney that may lead to nearly total loss of function. Pus may tract or form and perinephric abscess will form and can even burst in the loin, or a psoas abscess can form in the femoral triangle.

A5: What investigations would be most helpful and why?

- Full blood count (FBC), renal function and electrolytes
- Urine and blood cultures: most common organisms are coliforms (*Escherichia coli*, enterococci, *Proteus* spp., *Klebsiella* spp.)
- Ultrasonography: hydronephrosis, perinephric abscess
- Radiograph of the kidney, ureter and bladder: underlying stone
- CT urography: renal tract calcification and obstructing stones in the ureter

A6: What treatment options are appropriate?

Acute pyelonephritis is associated with fever and systemic symptoms for a shorter period and is treated with antibiotics. Imaging often rules out the presence of infected hydronephrosis or pyonephrosis/perinephric abscess. The antibiotics often work effectively within 4 to 5 days.

Impaired glomerular filtration inhibits the entry of antibiotics into the collecting system and requires emergency decompression by means of either percutaneous nephrostomy or ureteral stenting. The best course is treatment of sepsis and resuscitation as appropriate and urgent drainage of the kidney.

👥 OSCE Counselling cases

OSCE COUNSELLING CASE 5.2 – 'How do I prevent recurrent stone formation?'

- Increasing fluid intake, of up to 2 L per day, to maintain clear urine
- Animal protein restriction (reduced meat intake)
- Moderate calcium intake. Dietary calcium restriction actually increases stone recurrence risk by increase in the available intestinal oxalate. This increases intestinal oxalate absorption and supersaturation of calcium oxalate. Calcium supplementation is safest when taken with meals and calcium citrate is the safest and stone-friendly calcium supplement with the inhibitor action of citrate.
- Reduced-sodium diet

Obese patients may produce acidic urine and have increased incidence of uric acid stone formation. A low-carbohydrate, high-protein diet delivers a marked acid load to the kidney and increases risk of stone formation.

OSCE COUNSELLING CASE 5.3 – 'How do I counsel for extracorporeal shock wave lithotripsy (ESWL)?'

Extracorporeal shock wave lithotripsy is a non-invasive form of stone fragmentation achieved by directing shock waves onto the stone. Shock waves are generated by electrohydraulic, piezoelectric, electromagnetic sources, which are focused onto the ureteric or renal calculus, resulting in stone fragmentation. Stones are localized using radiographs or ultrasonography. A water-filled cushion in a silicone membrane provides the interface between the patient and the shock wave generator to minimize energy dissipation.

Acute UTIs, uncorrected bleeding disorders, pregnancy, sepsis and uncorrected obstruction distal to the stone are all considered absolute contraindications. Patients with cardiac and pulmonary problems are treated with caution. Dysrhythmias are common during lithotripsy and are controlled by cardiac gating. In this setting, the shock wave is discharged by the R wave in the cardiac cycle, which prevents most tachyrhythmias. Stone sizes >2 cm in diameter may require insertion of a JJ stent into the ureter to aid passage of stone fragments, and prevent the distal obstruction of the ureter from impacted stone fragments in the ureter – described as '*steinstrasse*' (stone street).

The stone fragmentation rate depends on the stone composition, stone size and position; calculi composed of calcium oxalate dihydrate, magnesium ammonium phosphate and uric acid fragment readily with ESWL. Calcium oxalate monohydrate and certain forms of calcium phosphate stones (e.g. brushite) are more difficult to fragment with ESWL and cystine stones are often resistant to such fragmentation. Stones within the lower pole calyx with an acute infundibulopelvic angle often do not clear, and this needs to be taken into consideration when offering advice.

The overall success rates are around 40 to 70 per cent.

The side effects of ESWL include pain, haematuria and loin bruising. Subcapsular haematomas in the perinephric region may be associated with severe loin pain and bruising, and may require parenteral opiates. Haematuria associated with stone fragmentation may present with clots. Pretreatment with 100 to 500 shocks at low energy levels to reduce lesion size and treatment at a slow rate of shock-wave delivery (60 shocks/min or less) reduce the risk of renal trauma with shock-wave lithotripsy.

The cardiac dysrhythmias may occur with previous cardiac abnormalities.

REVISION PANEL

- Ruptured abdominal aortic aneurysm is a differential diagnosis particularly in the older patient and may be identified by palpating pulsatile aneurysm in abdomen or urgent imaging.
- Loin pain may be associated with fever in pyelonephritis but also may be associated with infection in a closed renal unit. The presence of hydronephrosis in the context of sepsis with renal tenderness may require urgent drainage of the kidney with a nephrostomy or ureteric stenting.
- CT without contrast is the accepted gold standard investigation for suspected ureteric colic.
- Staghorn calculi may be asymptomatic or may have renal pain, recurrent urine infections or microscopic haematuria.
- Stones are often associated with infection and may require a multimodal approach to treat stones often requiring more than one treatment.
- Renal tract anatomy may be important to rule out coexisting abnormal anatomy.
- Obstructed kidney with sepsis leads to accelerated nephron loss. Infection in an obstructed kidney may lead to infected hydronephrosis or pyonephrosis. Treatment is drainage of the pus.
- Two factors differentiate pyonephrosis and acute pyelonephritis. Pyonephrosis is often associated with a prolonged period of fever prior to clinical presentation and often does not respond well to antibiotics alone and may require drainage.

BLADDER OUTFLOW OBSTRUCTION

Questions

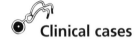

Clinical cases

For each of the clinical case scenarios given

> **Q1:** What is the likely differential diagnosis?
> **Q2:** What issues in the given history support/refute a particular diagnosis?
> **Q3:** What additional features would you seek to support a particular diagnosis?
> **Q4:** What clinical examination would you perform and why?
> **Q5:** What investigations would be most helpful and why?
> **Q6:** What treatment options are appropriate?

CASE 5.7 – 'My urine flow is poor'

A 64-year-old painter presents with a reduced urinary stream and incomplete emptying of the bladder with nocturia of two to three times a night. He is a smoker and has ischaemic heart disease.

CASE 5.8 – 'I am unable to pass urine'

72-year-old man presented with painful inability to pass urine after having much to drink at his daughter's wedding.

CASE 5.9 – 'My husband is confused and wet'

A lady presented with her 74-year-old husband who was increasingly confused and smelling of urine and wetting the bed.

OSCE Counselling case

OSCE COUNSELLING CASE 5.4 – **What are the effects of surgery on the prostate?**

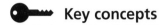 **Key concepts**

LOWER URINARY TRACT SYMPTOMS:

- Bladder outflow obstruction
- Benign prostatic enlargement
- BPH
- Acute urinary retention
- Acute or chronic urinary retention
- Chronic urinary retention
- Detrusor failure.

Answers

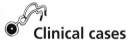
Clinical cases

CASE 5.7 – 'My urine flow is poor'

A1: What is the likely differential diagnosis?

- BPH
- Urethral stricture
- Prostatitis
- Prostate cancer

A2: What issues in the given history support/refute a particular diagnosis?

Lower urinary tract symptoms (LUTS) may be voiding in nature, when they present with hesitancy, reduced stream or interrupted stream. Voiding LUTS are often associated with bladder outflow obstruction but may also be due to detrusor failure. The diagnosis of BPH is histological in the prostate and is primarily obstructive but it also produces changes in bladder compliance that result in increased storage symptoms. Storage LUTS present with frequency of micturition, nocturia and urgency with or without urgency incontinence. The post-micturition LUTS are sensation of incomplete emptying and post-micturition dribble.

A3: What additional features would you seek to support a particular diagnosis?

- Aetiology: previous endoscopic procedures or infections, stone disease, family history of prostate cancer
- General fitness and quality of life: co-morbidity with ischaemic heart disease, hypertension, diabetes
- Scoring systems exist that would quantify the lower urinary tract dysfunction and the effect on the quality of life (i.e. international prostate symptom score [IPSS]). It also includes bothersomeness. This is important to determine treatment.

A4: What clinical examination would you perform and why?

Examination of the abdomen for a palpable bladder or masses and DRE to assess the size and consistency of the prostate are performed. Prostate tenderness is often associated with prostatitis.

A5: What investigations would be most helpful and why?

A frequency volume chart would be helpful as would urine dipstick, midstream urine (MSU) for culture and sensitivity, blood for serum creatinine, serum prostate-specific antigen (PSA) (if aged between 45 and 70 years and/or clinical examination suggests malignancy), urine flow rate and post-void residual volume of bladder by ultrasonography. Suspicious DRE or abnormal PSA must be appropriately investigated to rule out prostate cancer. Bladder or pelvic pain and neurological disease may need specialized investigations. Haematuria with lower urinary tract symptoms should be investigated as for haematuria.

A6: What treatment options are appropriate?

Conservative treatment: advice to all patients should be appropriate fluid intake; avoid caffeine or bladder stimulants and reduce intake of fluid after 8.00 p.m. Advise regarding bladder training.

Management depends on severity of symptoms (scored using an International Prostate Symptom Score [IPSS]) and bothersome LUTS. Voiding LUTS in patients with confirmed poor flow with a small-sized prostate may be treated with lifestyle and fluid advice, bladder retraining and alpha blockers. A larger prostate in the same group of patients may get added benefit from five alpha reductase inhibitors. PDE-5 inhibitors are shown to have similar efficacy in patients with voiding LUTS; there may be a role of treating patients with both erectile dysfunction (ED) and bladder outflow obstruction with PDE-5 inhibitors daily.

CASE 5.8 – 'I am unable to pass urine'

A1: What is the likely differential diagnosis?

- Obstruction to the urine outflow: prostatic enlargement
- Stress
- Neurological conditions: common in patients with multiple sclerosis and spinal cord compression (cauda equina lesion); consider this diagnosis in patients with associated abnormal neurology and in younger patients

A2: What issues in the given history support/refute a particular diagnosis?

History of previous obstructive lower urinary tract symptoms

A3: What additional features would you seek to support a particular diagnosis?

Triggers for acute urinary retention may be the following:

- Urine infection
- Alcohol intake
- Exacerbation of chronic obstructive airway and use of inhaled β-receptor agonists, or any drug with anticholinergic effects or α-adrenergic effects, such as antihistamines and ephedrine sulfate, which may precipitate retention
- Post-operative (major pelvic or orthopaedic surgery)
- Constipation
- Other conditions including genital herpes, urethral stone, prostatitis and haematuria with clot retention

Medical history of co-morbidity: diabetes, renal impairment.

Assess suitability for surgery and for α blockers (would cause postural hypotension, and judicious use is needed in elderly patients with compromised cardiovascular systems).

A4: What clinical examination would you perform and why?

- Confirm palpable bladder and abdominal examination to identify masses.
- Use DRE to identify masses in rectum and prostate assessment.
- Perform focused neurological examination including power and tendon reflexes in the legs and feet, examination for loss of sensation in the legs, feet and perineum. Test for anal tone, contraction of pelvic floor muscles and the presence of the bulbocavernosus reflex (tests the integrity of the sacral cord reflex, i.e. pudendal afferents, sacral segments S2–4 and pudendal efferents). This is seen as a reflex contraction of the pelvic floor on stimulation of the glans or clitoris. This may also be elicited by gently pulling the urethral catheter.

A5: What investigations would be most helpful and why?

- Catheter specimen of urine for microscopy and culture: UTI
- Serum creatinine: renal dysfunction caused by back pressure into the renal collecting system
- Ultrasonography of renal tract: assessment of kidneys

A6: What treatment options are appropriate?

- Initial treatment: symptomatic pain control, relief of retention with a urinary catheter may be provided.
- Medical treatment: there is a role for α blockers in acute urinary retention. This can be started and a trial without catheter may be given within 48 hours of starting the treatment. If this fails the options are either to proceed to surgery or to give another trial without a catheter in 2 weeks.
- Surgical treatment: the 'gold standard' procedure is a transurethral resection of the prostate (TURP). However, there are several other modalities of treatment including laser coagulation and enucleation that are being developed to achieve the same effect.

CASE 5.9 – 'My husband is confused and wet'

A1: What is the likely differential diagnosis?

Acute confusional state with incontinence:

- Diabetic acidosis, electrolyte abnormalities
- Infections and dehydration
- Cerebral metastasis
- Intracranial haemorrhage/cerebrovascular accident (CVA)

A2: What issues in the given history support/refute a particular diagnosis?

Gradually increasing confusion and urinary incontinence may be caused by urinary retention, with backpressure on the renal collecting system causing uraemia. Urinary tract infections or sepsis may lead to general deterioration of health and confusion with loss of control of bodily functions. Cerebrovascular accident or intracranial haemorrhage is associated with a neurological deficit.

A3: What additional features would you seek to support a particular diagnosis?

Chronic retention is a non-painful bladder that remains palpable or percussable after the patient has passed urine. Such patients may be incontinent. Chronic retention may occur in patients with detrusor underactivity, detrusor hyperactivity with impaired contractility or neurogenic bladder conditions and bladder outflow obstruction. Chronic urinary retention is generally classified as high-pressure and low-pressure chronic retention. The low-pressure group complained of hesitancy, slow stream and a feeling of incomplete emptying. The high-pressure group complained of urgency, and there is an association with upper tract dilatation and obstructive uropathy and raised creatinine.

A4: What clinical examination would you perform and why?

Clinical examination should be performed to identify palpable bladder, DRE for constipation, rectal lesions and assessment of prostate; also a focused neurological examination should be performed. Chronic retention may be associated with neurological disease and clinical examination may identify spinal cord compression or cauda equina lesion.

A5: What investigations would be most helpful and why?

- Urine dipstick and microscopy: to rule out infection
- U&Es: uraemia
- Ultrasonography to identify hydronephrosis and renal cortical thickness (long-standing hydronephrosis is associated with a thinning of the renal cortex)

A6: What treatment options are appropriate?

Catheterization in chronic retention has the risk of inducing sepsis, and decompression of urine and pressure in the renal collecting system are associated with haematuria and a post-obstructive diuresis. The haematuria may need to be treated with bladder washouts. It is important to correct the volume depleted as a result of diuresis to prevent a dehydration-induced/hypovolaemic acute tubular necrosis, in addition to the existing renal dysfunction.

OSCE Counselling case

OSCE COUNSELLING CASE 5.4 – **What are the effects of surgery on the prostate?**

Trans-urethral resection of the prostate is performed using a resectoscope through the urethra. It is commonly associated with post-operative bleeding, which is controlled with continuous bladder irrigation. The use of anticoagulants before the procedure increases the risk of bleeding.

Irrigating fluid (glycine) may be absorbed into the circulation, causing a trans-urethral resection syndrome with hypervolaemia and 1 to 3 per cent hyponatraemia. Mental confusion, nausea, vomiting and visual disturbance are noted, which are the result of fluid absorption and hyperammonaemia (glycine breaking down into ammonia and glycolic acid).

Surgery is associated with retrograde ejaculation in around 65 to 80 per cent of patients. The subsequent urine sample shows spermatozoa on microscopy.

There is conflicting evidence regarding erectile function, with either no change or some reduction in erectile function.

Failure to void after a TURP is present in up to 20 per cent of cases as a result of either insufficient resection of the prostate or detrusor failure.

Incontinence is rare (3 per cent) with urge and stress incontinence. Pre-existing detrusor overactivity caused by obstruction may manifest as urge incontinence and can be very distressing. Appropriate patient selection and counselling will reduce this risk. Resection close to the striated sphincter near the apex of the prostate may lead to sphincteric weakness, which manifests as stress incontinence or total incontinence. Conservative treatment with pelvic floor exercises may be helpful. An additional surgical procedure may be required to correct incontinence.

The alternatives are holmium laser enucleation of prostate (HoLEP) or laser ablation of the prostate (Green light laser).

REVISION PANEL

- Voiding LUTS, like hesitancy, poor flow and intermittency may be related to bladder outlet obstruction as a result of benign prostatic obstruction, which is often associated with benign prostatic enlargement (BPE). This may result from histological condition of BPH that is often within the transitional zone of the prostate.
- Failure to empty the bladder may be related to an outlet obstruction or to detrusor underactivity of the bladder or a combination of both.
- Acute urinary retention (AUR) is the most common urologic emergency managed by urologists worldwide. It is characterized by a sudden-onset, often painful inability to pass urine. It may be spontaneous where it is usually associated with previous voiding LUTS and when no precipitating causes are noted. Precipitated AUR is often related to medication (e.g. anticholinergic, UTI, excessive fluid intake, post-operative pain and regional anaesthesia).
- The presence of voiding LUTS, a low peak flow rate on voiding, prostatic enlargement and/or PSA increase are risk factors of AUR.
- Successful voiding after AUR is improved by using an alpha blocker at the time of AUR.
- The 5-alpha reductase inhibitors are shown to have a role in preventing risk of AUR or needing surgery. It is recommended in patients with risk factors for AUR but with minimal symptoms to start 5-alpha reductase inhibitors to reduce risk of AUR and subsequent AUR-related surgery.
- Chronic urinary retention (CUR) describes a bladder that does not empty completely or does not empty at all. It may be associated with either a high bladder pressure or low bladder pressure.
- The high-pressure CUR with detrusor muscle hypertrophy and associated urinary urgency may be associated with backpressure changes to the kidney and/or raised creatinine.
- The low-pressure CUR may be associated with bladder stones, overflow urinary incontinence, or urinary tract infections.
- Many studies suggest that patients benefit from disobstructive surgery with either a TURP or laser prostatectomy. Clean intermittent self-catheterization is also an option to empty the bladder and avoid surgery in low-pressure CUR.

PROSTATE CANCER AND PSA

Questions

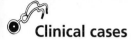

Clinical cases

For each of the clinical case scenarios given

Q1: What is the likely differential diagnosis?
Q2: What issues in the given history support/refute a particular diagnosis?
Q3: What additional features would you seek to support a particular diagnosis?
Q4: What clinical examination would you perform and why?
Q5: What investigations would be most helpful and why?
Q6: What treatment options are appropriate?

CASE 5.10 – 'I have a raised PSA of 4 ng/mL'

A 52-year-old businessman presents with a raised PSA after routine testing as part of his insurance screen. He is fit and well, and has no urinary symptoms.

CASE 5.11 – 'I have difficulty in passing urine'

A 73-year-old man presents with haematuria on and off, passed clots about 3 weeks ago which settled, and has difficulty passing urine, with hesitancy, nocturia and terminal dribbling.

CASE 5.12 – 'I have severe back pain and am "off my legs"'

An 82-year-old man from a nursing home was noted to be 'off his legs' and has been complaining of back pain for about 3 weeks. He has been losing weight over the last 3 months and has a reduced appetite.

👫 OSCE Counselling cases

OSCE COUNSELLING CASE 5.5 – **'Do I need a blood test to check for prostate cancer?'**

OSCE COUNSELLING CASE 5.6 – **'Will I be incontinent after my prostate operation?'**

Q1: What are the main complications of radical retropubic prostatectomy and will I be incontinent after a prostate operation?

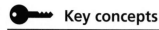 **Key concepts**

Prostate cancer is the most common cancer in the Western world and is one of the most common causes of death. The true incidence may be higher as postmortem studies show a higher incidence with increasing age with over 50 per cent of patients aged over 90 having prostate cancer, but few of these are clinically significant. The widespread use of prostate-specific antigen (PSA) is associated with an increased incidence of prostate cancer and also a stage shift towards earlier stages in detected cancers.

The higher the PSA level the more likely is the presence of prostate cancer. Large cancers can cause symptoms of bladder outflow obstruction. Prostate cancer may present with metastasis and spinal cord compression caused by vertebral metastases as a surgical emergency.

The Gleason grade for prostate cancer utilizes the architecture of the gland to describe the level of differentiation. Scores range from 1 to 5, with 1 being the least aggressive and 5 being the most aggressive. Prostate cancer is both heterogeneous and multifocal and the most predominant grade and the second-most predominant grade are added to make up the sum Gleason score (e.g. 3 + 2 = 5).

Treatment depends on the stage and grade of the tumour, and the co-morbidity of the patient.

Localized prostate cancer is often treated with an intention to cure. The decision to treat is based on the estimated life expectancy. The benefits of radical treatment take 5 to 10 years to become manifest and radical treatment is only offered if there is a 10-year life expectancy. The various options include radical prostatectomy (to remove the prostate), radical radiotherapy (external beam radiotherapy to prostate) or brachytherapy (installation of radioactive seeds into the prostate). In patients with a lower volume and no high-grade disease, it may be reasonable to actively monitor the cancer with a view to deferred radical treatment if there is progression of either the grade on repeat biopsies, stage on imaging or PSA progression.

Locally advanced, non-metastatic prostate cancer may be treated with radical radiotherapy along with 3 years of adjuvant anti-androgen therapy or anti-androgen treatment alone. Surgical removal of prostate cancer may also be considered in locally advanced disease with a risk of positive surgical margins that may be treated with adjuvant radiotherapy.

Metastatic prostate cancer is treated by anti-androgen therapy. Prostate cancer is testosterone dependent and castration therapy is associated with apoptosis. The circadian pattern of GnRH release in the body is altered by exogenous GnRH analogues at higher levels with continuous blood levels that initially cause an LH surge that results in a 'testosterone flare' or rise in testosterone followed by depletion of LH resulting in castrate levels of testosterone. Prostate cancer may progress following an initial response to castrate conditions by developing pathways to proliferate (castrate-resistant prostate cancer [CRPC]). There is a role for additional treatments like chemotherapy in this situation. The prognosis of CRPC is poor with average life expectancy of 18 months.

Answers

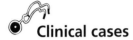

Clinical cases

CASE 5.10 – 'I have a raised PSA of 4 ng/mL'

A1: What is the likely differential diagnosis?

- BPH
- Prostate cancer
- Prostatitis
- UTI
- Prostatic calculi
- Instrumentation of the urethra and prostate

A raised PSA is not specific for prostate cancer but can occur with any of the above conditions and is prostate specific. The PSA levels in serum are related to the size of the prostate. The PSA may also increase with age and the age-specific PSA range in a man younger than 50 years is <2.5 ng/mL, whereas in a man >70 years PSA levels of up to 6.5 ng/mL are acceptable with low levels of prostate cancer. The incidence of prostate cancer diagnosis increases with raised baseline PSA levels at an early age. Compared to men with a baseline PSA of <1 ng/mL, higher levels of baseline PSA are associated with increased diagnosis of prostate cancer following a mean 28-year followup. There is a recommendation to do a baseline PSA at the age of 40 years and for 2-year follow-up if >1.0 ng/mL and if <1 ng/mL then to repeat this after 8 years.

A2: What issues in the given history support/refute a particular diagnosis?

There is no history of a previous UTI and urethral instrumentation or symptoms to suggest prostatitis. Prostate cancer needs to be excluded.

A3: What additional features would you seek to support a particular diagnosis?

Urinary symptoms suggest a urinary infection and symptoms of prostatitis. Risk factors of prostate cancer include family history, age and race (more common in men of African/Caribbean origin and less common in Asian men).

A4: What clinical examination would you perform and why?

Clinical examination should include a DRE to assess the prostate. A tender prostate would suggest prostatitis. The presence of a nodule or hard lobe of the prostate suggests a cancer. Digital rectal examination is also useful to assess local spread to the seminal vesicles and laterally beyond the prostate in advanced disease.

A5: What investigations would be most helpful and why?

- Urine microscopy isolates urine infection.
- Repeat PSA is more useful in borderline elevations and also in the presence of urine infection, prostatitis or recent instrumentation.
- Urine tumour marker (PCA3) after collecting initial urine sample following prostatic massage may add diagnostic value to PSA.

- Transrectal ultrasonography is useful to identify abnormal anatomy of the prostate and also to target prostate biopsies.
- Prostate biopsy is the gold standard for making a diagnosis.
- A bone scan would be useful to identify bony metastases if the PSA is >10 ng/mL.

A6: What treatment options are appropriate?

Localized prostate cancer   Treatment options are radical prostatectomy, radical radiotherapy, brachytherapy and active surveillance.

Reasons for a radical prostatectomy
- It removes a potential source of metastatic and locally advanced disease.
- Early prostate cancers allow for a nerve-sparing prostatectomy with preservation of potency.
- It removes a gland that grows with age and may eventually cause lower urinary tract symptoms.
- Early assessment of cure can be made with PSA measurements (which should be zero).
- Use of salvage radiotherapy is effective, safe and well established in cases of failure. Surgery after radiotherapy is possible although far less well established.
- There is no risk of second malignancy.
- The keyhole (laparoscopic) approach is minimally invasive.

Reasons for radical radiotherapy/brachytherapy   It has comparable results to radical surgery. External beam radiotherapy is focused radiation to the prostate delivered in daily fraction to achieve the cumulative radiation dosage. Brachytherapy involves implantation of radioactive seeds into the prostate.

Reasons for choosing active monitoring   In lower-grade tumours with small-volume disease it may be reasonable to monitor them closely with frequent PSA measurements and to treat aggressively if evidence of disease or grade progression is noted.

- High-grade prostatic intraepithelial neoplasia (PIN): this may be a pre-neoplastic condition and also suggests that there is adjacent prostate cancer; a repeat biopsy is recommended. Close observation is prudent.
- Normal biopsy: The PSA needs to be monitored because there is a risk of a false-negative biopsy as a result of a sampling error; a rising PSA would necessitate further investigation (repeat prostate biopsies).

CASE 5.11 – 'I have difficulty in passing urine'

A1: What is the likely differential diagnosis?
- BPH
- Prostate cancer
- Urethral stricture

A2: What issues in the given history support/refute a particular diagnosis?

The patient presents with local symptoms of urinary outflow obstruction. Family history of prostate cancer is a known risk factor for prostate cancer.

A3: What additional features would you seek to support a particular diagnosis?

Prostate cancer may be locally advanced with urinary obstruction and may present with haematuria. Locally advanced prostate cancer may also involve the trigone of the bladder and obstruct one or both ureters, causing hydronephrosis and uraemia. Metastatic prostate cancer spreads to bones and lymph nodes. The presence of bony pain and nodal enlargement is elicited.

A4: What clinical examination would you perform and why?

Clinical examination to identify the presence of a palpable bladder and DRE to identify the stage of the prostate cancer should be performed.

A5: What investigations would be most helpful and why?

- Urine microscopy: rule out infection or prostatitis
- PSA: >15 ng/mL is associated with an increased risk of metastatic prostatic cancer
- U&Es: uraemia
- Transrectal ultrasonography and prostate biopsy: confirm diagnosis of prostate cancer
- Ultrasonography of renal tract: hydronephrosis and renal cortex thickness
- Bone scan: to identify bone metastasis

A6: What treatment options are appropriate?

Symptomatic prostate cancer is treated on the basis of being clinically localized or metastatic. Clinically localized disease is treated with radical treatment (i.e. surgery, radiotherapy or active surveillance). Brachytherapy is not suitable for patients with lower urinary tract symptoms because subsequent transurethral surgery has a high risk of incontinence or if the prostate volume is >40 cc.

Locally advanced prostate cancer may be treated symptomatically. Bladder outflow obstruction may be treated with hormones if there are no signs of urinary retention. Hormone treatment is known to reduce the size of the prostate and will improve the urinary symptoms. Hormone treatment may be followed by surgery or radiotherapy in selected patients.

Intermittent hormone treatment is being considered and has the advantage of a 'treatment holiday' to improve the quality of life of patients on hormone therapy/androgen withdrawal without affecting survival.

CASE 5.12 – 'I have severe back pain and am "off my legs"'

A1: What is the likely differential diagnosis?

- Spinal cord compression from tumour or osteoporotic collapse
- Subdural or epidural abscess or haematoma
- Transverse myelitis
- Multiple sclerosis (MS)
- Acute postviral – Guillain-Barré disease

A2: What issues in the given history support/refute a particular diagnosis?

- Pain in the back or radiating from the back – can be exacerbated by coughing or movement. This is the most common symptom in up to 75 per cent of patients and precedes neurological symptoms. Pain may be focal, radicular or referred.
- Weakness and loss of sensation in lower part of the body, sensation loss helps identify spinal level of cord compression
- Retention of urine
- Bowel and bladder dysfunction: urinary retention or urinary incontinence (overflow or stress leak due to sphincter incompetence)
- Fecal incontinence

A3: What additional features would you seek to support a particular diagnosis?

A sequence of events with pain, loss of function and loss of sensation should be sought. The pain and mild weakness may last hours to days, but the transition to total loss of function distal to the lesion may take only minutes.

Patients who are started on hormone treatment with androgen withdrawal (GnRH analogues) have a 'testosterone flare' resulting from the initial stimulation of the testosterone release by the GnRH release; this must be monitored carefully because it may induce an enlargement of the spinal metastasis and precipitate cord compression. Therefore, it is important to use an anti-androgen for 2 weeks before the GnRH injection. Involvement of the spine is due to local extension of the vertebral metastases. Tumour compression leads to venous congestion/obstruction and vasogenic oedema. This local oedema may respond to steroids.

A4: What clinical examination would you perform and why?

- Examination of the abdomen and DRE
- Focused neurological examination necessary to identify cord compression
- Spine tenderness (percussion tenderness is especially prominent with metastatic carcinoma, vertebral infection, or spinal or epidural abscess), paraparesis, sensory deficits of the limbs or trunk, and corticospinal reflex changes

A5: What investigations would be most helpful and why?

- PSA
- Transrectal ultrasonography and prostate biopsy: diagnose prostate cancer
- Plain spinal radiograph: identifies sclerosis, osteoporosis and crush fractures
- CT or magnetic resonance imaging (MRI) of spine: tumours in spine with cord compression and nerve root involvement. MRI is now the gold standard investigation for spinal cord compression. It is useful in diagnosing extra-dural metastasis, intramedullary lesions, vertebral lesions and paravertebral lesions.

A6: What treatment options are appropriate?

Any patient with suspected spinal cord compression should be admitted as an emergency for investigation and treatment. Once paralysed, only 5 per cent walk again; 30 per cent of patients survive to 1 year.

The best results are obtained when treatment is instituted early:

- Medical treatment: dexamethasone to relieve the oedema, analgesia
- Radiotherapy: useful to reduce the compression urgently
- Surgery: surgical decompression, urgent referral to a neurosurgeon

👥 OSCE Counselling case

OSCE COUNSELLING CASE 5.5 – 'Do I need a blood test to check for prostate cancer?'

If the PSA is elevated the risk of having prostate cancer depends on the value:

- PSA 4 to 10: risk of underlying prostate cancer is 25 per cent
- PSA >10: risk of underlying prostate cancer is 50 per cent

The probability (percentage) of prostate cancer depends on age and DRE (Table 5.1).

A prostate biopsy has a 1 to 3 per cent risk of complications of bleeding, infection and urinary retention. A prostate cancer prevention trial (PCPT) was reported in 2004 with 18 882 men enrolled in the prevention trial, 9459 were randomly assigned to receive placebo and had an annual measurement of PSA and a DRE. Among these 9459 men, 2950 men never had a PSA level of more than 4 ng/mL or an abnormal DRE, had a final PSA determination, and underwent a prostate biopsy after being in the study for 7 years. Among the 2950 men (age range, 62 to 91 years), prostate cancer was diagnosed in 449 (15.2 per cent); 67 of these 449 cancers (14.9 per cent) had a Gleason score of 7 or higher. The prevalence of prostate cancer was 6.6 per cent among men with a PSA level of up to 0.5 ng/mL, 10.1 per cent among those with values of 0.6 to 1 ng/mL, 17 per cent among those with values of 1.1 to 2 ng/mL, 23.9 per cent among those with values of 2.1 to 3 ng/mL, and 26.9 per cent among those with values of 3.1 to 4 ng/mL. The prevalence of high-grade cancers increased from 12.5 per cent of cancers associated with a PSA level of 0.5 ng/mL or less to 25 per cent of cancers associated with a PSA level of 3.1 to 4 ng/mL.

Table 5.1 PSA Score and DRE Result

Age (years)	<50		51–60		61–70		71–80	
PSA (ng/mL)	DRE–	DRE+	DRE–	DRE+	DRE–	DRE+	DRE–	DRE+
<2.5	9	37	12	39	15	42	20	44
2.6–4.0	9	41	12	42	16	44	20	47
4.1–6.0	10	41	14	44	17	47	22	48
6.1–10.0	11	13	15	48	19	50	25	42
10.1–20.0	13	55	19	54	25	58	31	60
>20.0	22	82	45	74	43	81	59	84

Note: DRE, digital rectal examination; PSA, prostate-specific antigen; DRE–, normal DRE; DRE+, abnormal DRE.
Source: Data from Potter et al., *Urology* 57, 1100–1104, 2001; and Thompson et al., *N Engl J Med* 350, 2239–2246, 2004.

Benefits of PSA testing

1. It may provide reassurance if the test result is normal.
2. It may find cancer before symptoms develop.
3. It may detect cancer at an early stage when treatments could be beneficial.
4. If treatment is successful, the consequences of more advanced cancers are avoided.
5. Screening might detect the cancer at an earlier stage. Increasing evidence shows that most screen-detected cancers will never kill and that the subset of lethal PCa probably has a much shorter lead time and benefits from earlier detection and treatment.

There are currently no tests to identify patients that are more likely to progress once detected and active surveillance with an intention to cure but offering deferred radical treatment at progression is a reasonable option to minimize the problem of overtreatment/side effects related to radical therapy.

Downside of PSA testing

1. It can miss cancer and provide false reassurance.
2. It may lead to unnecessary anxiety and medical tests when no cancer is present.
3. It might detect slow-growing cancer that may never cause any symptoms or shorten life span.
4. The main treatments of prostate cancer have significant side effects, and there is some overtreatment of patients due to screening for prostate cancer. There was a 21 per cent mortality reduction reported at 11 years of follow-up in the core age group of the European randomized screening study for prostate cancer (ERSPC) that was achieved in men who entered at an age between 55 and 69 years. The numbers needed to screen and then treat to avoid one prostate cancer–related death were 837 and 29 at 10 years and 503 and 18 at 12 years, respectively.

Routine PSA screening is not currently recommended in the United Kingdom for asymptomatic individuals. However, the PSA test may be performed in patients aged over 50 years who present with lower urinary tract symptoms or who request it.

Those with a family history of prostate cancer and from an African-Caribbean origin should be advised to be tested from the age of 40 years as a baseline value and if the level is <1 ng/mL then further tests may be repeated in 8 years and if >1 ng/mL then may be repeated in 2 years.

OSCE COUNSELLING CASE 5.6 – 'Will I be incontinent after my prostate operation?'

Q1: What are the main complications of radical retropubic prostatectomy and will I be incontinent after a prostate operation?

Surgery is commonly offered to patients with an expected survival of over 10 years and localized prostate cancer.

Surgery may be performed by an open or laparoscopic/robotic route: the open approach may be retropubic or perineal. A bilateral nerve-sparing approach may be considered if suitable; this is more likely to preserve erectile function. A laparoscopic/robotic route has the advantage of minimum morbidity with equivalent oncological outcomes.

Inpatient stay varies with the approach used: open operations require a stay of 4 to 7 days and the laparoscopic route requires 2 to 4 days.

The following are the common complications:

*   Impotence: where bilateral nerve sparing is performed the return of erectile function is between 50 and 70 per cent. Bilateral nerve sparing is only safely offered to patients with early disease (i.e. screen detected). Taking all types of radical prostatectomy together (i.e. nerve and non-nerve-sparing), recent studies suggest that over 56 per cent of men will be completely impotent and a further 29 per cent will have a reduced erection.
*   Incontinence: severe incontinence is noted in 1 to 3 per cent, and occasional loss of control in 10 to 20 per cent of patients.
*   Mortality: the mortality rate is 0.7 per cent.

REVISION PANEL

- PSA is prostate specific and not cancer specific, age-specific PSAs are currently used to define normal values. PSA increases with age and other variables like PSA density (PSA in comparison to the volume of the prostate), PSA velocity (rise in PSA over time) and PSA doubling time (time taken for PSA to double is a variable that helps in prostate cancer diagnosis and management of patients with raised PSA).
- Baseline values of PSA at the age of 40 years may help predict future risk of prostate cancer diagnosis. A lower baseline value of <1 ng/mL may need to be repeated in 8 years, while a baseline value at the age of 40 years of >1 ng/mL may need to be monitored more closely and repeated in 2 years.
- Widespread use of PSA has led to reduction in the incidence of metastatic prostate cancer, but it has also led to the use of increased widespread use of radical treatments for prostate cancer, often resulting in overtreatment.
- Population-based screening for prostate cancer using PSA is not yet recommended as the benefits are not fully demonstrated. The screening has shown to reduce mortality but at the cost of overtreatment.
- Prostate cancer may present with lower urinary tract symptoms, symptoms of obstructive uropathy by trigone involvement and also by metastatic cancer with bone pain and/or spinal cord compression.
- Localized prostate cancer is managed by radical treatment or surveillance with an intention for deferred radical treatment with disease progression (active surveillance). Radical treatment may involve either removing the prostate (radical prostatectomy) or radiotherapy to the prostate (external beam radiotherapy or installation of radioactive seeds into the prostate – brachytherapy).
- Locally advanced prostate cancer is often treated using radical radiotherapy with adjuvant hormone treatment. Radical surgery may be offered in some cases of locally advanced disease but is often supported by adjuvant radiotherapy for positive surgical margins.
- Metastatic prostate cancer is treated by medical castration therapy and often responds by demonstrating a PSA response and clinical response by reduction of pain. Following an initial response the prostate cancer often progresses despite castration into a castrate-resistant prostate cancer.
- Metastatic prostate cancer with spinal cord compression is a common neurological complication of advanced malignancy and should be considered an oncological emergency.
- Patients present with back pain that precedes spinal cord compression, other features include weakness and sensory loss in lower limbs and urinary retention/incontinence.
- The gold standard investigation to identify spinal cord compression is MRI and aggressive investigation of patients with suspected spinal cord compression and urgent treatment leads to best outcomes.
- Confirmation of diagnosis and dexamethasone to reduce oedema and decompression either surgically or by radiotherapy of the lesion in the spine rapidly allow for improved outcomes.

INCONTINENCE

Questions

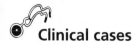
Clinical cases

For each of the clinical case scenarios given

Q1: What is the likely differential diagnosis?
Q2: What issues in the given history support/refute a particular diagnosis?
Q3: What additional features would you seek to support a particular diagnosis?
Q4: What clinical examination would you perform and why?
Q5: What investigations would be most helpful and why?
Q6: What treatment options are appropriate?

CASE 5.13 – 'I have a urinary leak every time I cough or strain'

A 48-year-old woman is postmenopausal and has a minor leak of urine every time she coughs and sneezes. She has three children, the last one needing a forceps delivery.

CASE 5.14 – 'I can't get to the toilet in time'

A 24-year-old teacher notes frequency and urgency every 30 minutes and urge incontinence.

CASE 5.15 – 'I have been leaking ever since the operation'

A 38-year-old woman has been continually wet after a vaginal hysterectomy. She did not have any urinary symptoms before the operation.

⚇ OSCE Counselling case

OSCE COUNSELLING CASE 5.7 – 'I keep going to the toilet every 30 minutes!'

A 34-year-old solicitor has difficulty coping with work because she has to go to the toilet every 30 minutes; she has daytime frequency and urgency and no nocturia. She has recurrent episodes of cystitis although the urine tests do not grow any organisms. She takes 10 cups of tea every day and about three to four cans of coke. She has no children. She had a normal bladder examination and biopsy.

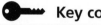 **Key concepts**

- Urinary incontinence: involuntary leakage of urine
- Urodynamic stress incontinence (USI), previously called genuine stress incontinence

    USI is noted during filling cystometry, and is defined as the involuntary leakage of urine during increased abdominal pressure in the absence of a detrusor contraction. This is caused by a failure to maintain the normal retropubic position of the bladder neck and posterior urethra during increases in abdominal pressure and/or impaired internal sphincter mechanism.

    - Detrusor overactivity, previously called detrusor instability

        Detrusor overactivity is a urodynamic observation characterized by involuntary detrusor contractions during the filling phase which may be spontaneous or provoked.

- An overactive bladder is a symptom complex that includes urinary urgency with or without urge incontinence, urinary frequency (voiding eight or more times in a 24-hour period) and nocturia (awakening two or more times at night to void). It is a syndrome with no precise cause and local causes are excluded. The urodynamic evidence of detrusor overactivity is commonly noted in patients with an overactive bladder.

    Patients with symptoms of an overactive bladder with underlying mucosal (carcinoma in situ, interstitial cystitis, cystitis, bladder stone) or neurological causes (Parkinson's disease, MS, spinal cord injury, diabetic neuropathy) and extrinsic causes (e.g. bladder outlet obstruction) are excluded from the overactive bladder syndrome. The urodynamic diagnosis is confirmed by detrusor overactivity in the filling phase of urodynamics.

- Total incontinence may be a result of complete loss of sphincteric control or a fistula (abnormal communication between the urinary tract and the skin). The most common cause of fistulae is iatrogenic and may be ureterovaginal or vesicovaginal.

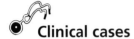

Answers

Clinical cases

CASE 5.13 – 'I have a urinary leak every time I cough or strain'

A1: What is the likely differential diagnosis?

- USI, most likely
- Detrusor overactivity (urge incontinence)
- Mixed incontinence (USI and detrusor overactivity)
- Overflow incontinence resulting from neurological causes or anticholinergic effects of drugs
- UTI
- Atrophic vaginitis/menopausal symptoms
- Acute confusional state
- Increased urine output (e.g. heart failure, diuretics, hyperglycaemia)

A2: What issues in the given history support/refute a particular diagnosis?

Urodynamic stress incontinence is more common in patients who are post-menopausal or post-child-bearing. This is commonly attributed to weakening of the pelvic floor muscles and loss of anterior vaginal support of the urethra to allow optimal closure mechanism.

A3: What additional features would you seek to support a particular diagnosis?

- Lower urinary tract symptoms would be in keeping with an overactive bladder such as frequency, urgency, nocturia or suprapubic discomfort.
- Voiding diary would be used to identify the amount and type of fluid intake and the frequency of voiding with urinary leaks. The number of pads and pad weight (as a measure of severity of leakage) could be assessed.
- The causes of an abnormal urethral support mechanism include congenital weakness and shortness of the vagina, difficult labour, multiparity and menopause. Iatrogenic causes include radical or simple hysterectomy and other types of extensive pelvic surgery.
- Oestrogen deficiency plays a role in the maintenance of the pliability of the urethral mucosa and submucosa and may also present with dyspareunia.
- Chronic inflammatory tissue from previous surgical procedures and radiotherapy also compromises the urethral closure mechanism.
- The sphincteric weakness resulting from damage to the innervation of the urethral musculature may also lead to stress urinary leak: sensory loss and history of neurological dysfunction.

A4: What clinical examination would you perform and why?

- A clinical diagnosis of stress incontinence is often made by good history and examination and further testing with urodynamics is usually not necessary except for surgical considerations. The absence of urgency symptoms and complete bladder emptying and demonstrable stress leak on straining often help in diagnosis.
- Focused neurological examination should be performed including examination of power and tendon reflexes of the legs and feet, and examination for loss of sensation in legs, feet and perineum. Bulbocavernosus reflex and anal tone are also performed.

- Descent of the pelvic floor and anterior vaginal wall is noted with a Valsalva manoeuvre. Loss of urine when the bladder is partially full, and eradication of this leak when the urethra is supported by digital elevation of the urethrovesical junction, suggest that surgical correction would be effective.
- Assessment of the contraction of the pelvic floor muscles, pelvic prolapse and the oestrogen status in the vagina should be assessed.

A5: What investigations would be most helpful and why?

- Urine dipstick and urine culture should be performed to rule out urine infection.
- Postvoid residual measurement helps to identify the treatment procedure and whether further investigations are necessary.
- Women with pure stress incontinence in the absence of storage voiding LUTS and good bladder emptying often do not require further urodynamics. However, many women have mixed symptoms with/or bladder emptying difficulties and urodynamics helps define bladder function in this situation.
- Valsalva leak-point pressure and fluoroscopy may rarely be performed and are useful for identifying the anatomy of the bladder neck and urethra.

A6: What treatment options are appropriate?

Behaviour and physical therapy   All patients benefit from behavioural therapy which includes education to understand their condition and develop strategies to reduce incontinence.

- Fluid and dietary advice, smoking cessation, urge avoidance and reinforcement and timed voiding and 3-day bladder diary.
- Pelvic floor muscle training
- Use of vaginal cones with weights, vaginal electrical stimulation and biofeedback

Pharmacotherapy   α-Adrenergic agonists act on the bladder neck and proximal urethra and increase the urethral closure pressure (e.g. ephedrine, phenylpropanolamine).

Another agent, duloxetine, which is a dual serotonin (5-HT)/noradrenaline (norepinephrine) re-uptake blocker with antidepressant action, is also useful in stress incontinence but its use is restricted due to side effects.

Tricyclic antidepressants, which inhibit the re-uptake of noradrenaline, and their anticholinergic effects simultaneously inhibit bladder activity and are useful in mixed incontinence.

Surgery   Urodynamic stress incontinence caused by urethral hypermobility and descent of the bladder neck may be assessed clinically and correction of the abnormality is sufficient to improve symptoms.

Tension-free vaginal tape placement and colposuspension are useful in correcting urethral hypermobility and have good long-term effects.

CASE 5.14 – 'I can't get to the toilet in time'

A1: What is the likely differential diagnosis?

- Detrusor overactivity
- Ingestion of bladder stimulants (e.g. caffeine, alcohol etc.)
- Cystitis
- Bladder abnormalities (e.g. bladder stone, interstitial cystitis, bladder cancer)
- Obstruction (e.g. in men with prostate enlargement)
- Neurological conditions: stroke, MS
- Increased urine output (e.g. diabetes, cardiac failure)

A2: What issues in the given history support/refute a particular diagnosis?

Increased fluid intake and bladder stimulants are one of the most common causes of increased urinary frequency and urgency. A bladder diary often helps to identify the volume of fluid intake, type of fluids ingested and void volumes and intervals of voiding and incontinence episodes.

A3: What additional features would you seek to support a particular diagnosis?

A voiding diary (frequency and volume of voiding including incontinence episodes) and fluid volume chart (record of the amount and type of fluid intake) are crucial to the diagnosis.

An overactive bladder is usually urgency associated with urinary frequency and often nocturia with or without urinary urge incontinence.

A4: What clinical examination would you perform and why?

- Examination to rule out a palpable bladder, neurological examination
- Assessment of the contraction of the pelvic floor muscles, pelvic prolapse and the vaginal oestrogen status
- Assessment of the prostate in men by DRE.

A5: What investigations would be most helpful and why?

- Urine dipstick and microscopy: exclude cystitis
- Blood glucose and electrolytes: diabetes and renal impairment
- Urine cytology: useful screen for bladder cancer
- Cystoscopy and/or biopsy: interstitial cystitis and carcinoma in situ identified with a bladder biopsy and appearance on cystoscopy
- Ultrasonography and radiograph: postvoid residual volume, assessment of kidneys and screen for bladder calculi
- Flow rate (in men)
- Urodynamics: diagnose detrusor overactivity

A6: What treatment options are appropriate?

Behavioural modification   Weight reduction, fluid advice (avoid bladder stimulants, moderate intake), timid voiding and urge inhibition are encouraged.

Pelvic floor training has been shown to be effective in management of overactive bladder. Biofeedback and electrical stimulation are also useful adjuncts to treatment.

Pharmacotherapy   Anticholinergics acting on the muscarinic receptors are useful to suppress involuntary bladder contractions. The common side effects include dry mouth, constipation and blurred vision, which can be troublesome. Beta-3 agonists are the newest addition to the treatment of overactive bladder.

Tricyclic antidepressants also have similar effects on the bladder and often a combination may be required.

Surgery
- Cystoscopy and biopsy are useful to rule out inflammatory causes of overactive bladder symptoms.
- Cystoscopic injection of Botox® into the bladder has been shown to have significantly improved refractory overactive bladder.
- Augmentation of the bladder using a patch of detubularized bowel or by a detrusor myomectomy has been used.

- Extradural stimulation of the S3 nerve root exerts its effect by stimulating the sacral sensory fibres, which have the ability to inhibit the sacral parasympathetic neurons responsible for detrusor contraction.

CASE 5.15 – 'I have been leaking ever since the operation'

A1: What is the likely differential diagnosis?
- Vesicovaginal fistula/ureterovaginal fistula
- Urethral incontinence

A2: What issues in the given history support/refute a particular diagnosis?
- History of operation, no urinary symptoms before surgery affect the diagnosis.
- Iatrogenic trauma is the most common cause of fistulae in developed countries. Obstructed labour is the most common cause in the developing world.

A3: What additional features would you seek to support a particular diagnosis?
- The type of operation is important to the aetiology: abdominal hysterectomy, Wertheim's hysterectomy, anterior colporrhaphy or vaginal hysterectomy. The risk of ureteric injury after a standard hysterectomy is 0.5 to 1.5 per cent and the risk of a fistula is <1 per cent. The fistula develops soon after the procedure or may be delayed by 2 or more weeks if ischaemic necrosis of the tissues is its cause.
- History of irradiation is an important cause of genitourinary fistulae. They are associated with bladder pain and infection in 40 per cent of cases.
- Direct invasion in late stages of cancer (e.g. cervical cancer) is seen.
- The severity of urine loss by number of pads and pad weight is assessed.

A4: What clinical examination would you perform and why?
- Examine the abdomen and genitalia and note radiation changes and dermatitis from urinary contact of the skin.
- Perform a three-pad test by inserting three dry cotton-wool swabs into the upper, middle and lower thirds of the vagina. The bladder is adequately distended with methylene blue and any leakage around the catheter is stopped. The swabs in the lower and middle third of the vagina soaking with methylene blue would indicate a vesicovaginal fistula. If the upper third vaginal swab is soaked with clear urine it is likely to be a uretrovaginal fistula (multiple fistulae and vesicouretric reflux may yield false-positive results).
- Directly inspect the vagina after instillation of dye into the bladder to see the size and site of the fistula.

A5: What investigations would be most helpful and why?
- Biochemical analysis of the fluid is conducted to confirm urine leak.
- IVU: ureteric fistula is associated with ureteric dilatation and/or hydronephrosis and extravasation of contrast. To assist in delineating anatomy of the lower urinary tract MRI or CT urography may be used.
- Cystoscopy and examination under anaesthetic may be helpful to assess the pliability of the tissues and define the fistula.

A6: What treatment options are appropriate?
Initially insert a catheter and often a small fistula will heal in 3 to 4 weeks by conservative management.

Surgical repair may become necessary and often the first operation is the best chance to cure the patient, so it must be done by an expert in a specialist centre with appropriate support.

Early repair is in favour because of the improvement in quality of life. If injury to the bladder or ureter is noted intraoperatively, it must be repaired immediately. However, commonly the fistula is not obvious until 2 to 3 weeks after the procedure. The urine needs to be diverted with either a catheter or a nephrostomy as necessary and the infection treated.

The basic principles of fistula repair are as follows:

- The fistulous tract is excised to healthy, well-vascularized tissue.
- The repair should be tension free and multilayered using absorbable sutures.
- Techniques to improve the viability of the tissue by interposing well-vascularized tissues between the bladder and vagina (e.g. a Martius flap using a flap of labial fibrofatty tissue and the omental flap) are used.

ii OSCE Counselling case

OSCE COUNSELLING CASE 5.7 – 'I keep going to the toilet every 30 minutes!'

Urodynamics showed that catheterization was painful. It shows a reduced first sensation of filling and a reduced bladder capacity as a result of discomfort. There was no detrusor overactivity or rise in the detrusor pressure during filling.

The patient is worried that she will require major surgery. Counsel her about the various options available.

Bladder filling/storage failure

This may be caused by detrusor overactivity that may be idiopathic. It may also be caused in the absence of detrusor overactivity as in this case. This occurs due to increased afferent input from inflammation, irritation and causes of hypersensitivity of the bladder and bladder pain. Increased afferent activity may result from urgency without detrusor activity. The diurnal severity of symptoms is typical of afferent sensory pathway activation.

The treatment for a hypersensitive bladder (increased bladder sensation during filling the bladder at urodynamics) is treatment of the cause of the condition, which is often cystitis, urethritis, inflammatory bladder conditions such as interstitial cystitis, post-irradiation cystitis, or chemical or cyclophosphamide cystitis.

The treatment is to maintain a voiding diary and a fluid volume chart. Reduction in bladder stimulants such as tea and cola would help to improve symptoms. Bladder retraining, use of pelvic floor exercises and biofeedback techniques have a role in management. The involvement of the patient in self-help groups and judicious use of anticholinergics are useful.

Surgery has a minor role.

REVISION PANEL

- Urodynamic stress incontinence is diagnosed by a good history of leaking with straining, usually has good bladder emptying and no urgency or storage LUTS. Urodynamics is often not necessary to make this diagnosis but is confirmatory.
- Stress leak is quantified by 3-day voiding diary and pad testing. Various questionnaires help to assess quality of life impairment. Physical examination and bladder emptying are helpful in making diagnosis.
- The treatment of stress urinary incontinence is by fluid management, behavioural techniques, pelvic floor training followed by surgery to reinforce the anterior vaginal wall support to the urethra to effectively improve the closure mechanism.
- Overactive bladder (OAB) is a symptom complex and the urodynamic investigation often is associated with detrusor overactivity.
- OAB is often classified as dry OAB and wet OAB based on the presence of urgency incontinence. Bladder function and emptying are important and quantified by a 3-day bladder diary and pad testing. Questionnaires are helpful to identify quality of life impairment.
- The management is often pharmacotherapy to either reduce the muscarinic output to the bladder or beta-adrenergic therapy.
- Refractory OAB is often treated with surgical treatment options (e.g. Botox injections, sacral neuromodulation).
- Total incontinence may be due to sphincteric loss (urethral incontinence) or extra urethral loss (extra-anatomic loss of urine due to fistula).
- Extra-urethral loss of urine is often diagnosed by contrast imaging studies.
- In early stages (6 weeks and under) it is best to have a primary repair of the fistula; in later stages it is reasonable to effect urinary drainage to ensure the fistula site is healed and well vascularized and dry followed by delayed repair.

NEUROPATHIC BLADDER

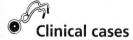

Clinical cases

For each of the clinical case scenarios given

> **Q1:** What is the likely differential diagnosis?
> **Q2:** What issues in the given history support/refute a particular diagnosis?
> **Q3:** What additional features would you seek to support a particular diagnosis?
> **Q4:** What clinical examination would you perform and why?
> **Q5:** What investigations would be most helpful and why?
> **Q6:** What treatment options are appropriate?

CASE 5.16 – 'I have leakage and have to go very frequently'

A 30-year-old T6 paraplegic woman has been performing intermittent self-catheterization (ISC) for 3 years since her accident. She has been on maximum doses of anticholinergics and has been leaking in between her catheterizations. She also notices pain in her loin, recurrent infections and one episode of pyelonephritis. Q1 is not applicable in this case.

CASE 5.17 – 'I am unable to pass urine'

A 35-year-old woman presented with inability to pass urine, and had loss of power and a tingling sensation in her feet. She also noticed constipation in the last 2 weeks and burning sensation over her genitalia. She had an episode of transient blurring of the vision in her right eye but recovered spontaneously about 2 years ago.

CASE 5.18 – 'I have recurrent infections'

A 27-year-old who was paraplegic after a road traffic accident has been performing ISC for about 3 years and presents with increasing UTIs. Over the last 6 months he has had over six infections. Q1 is only applicable.

Key concepts

- Spinal cord injury
- Sacral/cauda equina lesion
- Detrusor-sphincter dyssynergia (DSD)

The storage phase in the bladder accounts for most of its function. This is maintained by inhibition of the parasympathetic activity (sacral spinal cord) that leads to active relaxation of the detrusor. The sphincter is contracted by sympathetic and pudendal nerves at this phase of bladder function to maintain continence. The voiding phase is initiated by sensory output from the bladder that causes micturition reflex. This leads to inhibition of the pudendal nerve and suppression of sympathetic activity and active contraction of the detrusor. Three voiding centres control bladder function. The sacral micturition centre (S2, 3, 4) controls both the parasympathetic (detrusor output) and pudendal (sphincteric output). The pontine micturition centre in the midbrain coordinates the two sacral areas to relax sphincters and contract detrusor and vice versa. The third control centre is in the voluntary control of micturition in the cerebral cortex that initiates or delays voiding depending on social circumstances.

The possible dysfunctions that occur may either be a failure to store or failure to empty. The most common symptom is that of the former and incontinence. Some may have a combination with incomplete emptying and bladder overactivity, particularly those with spinal cord disease. Spinal cord disease is also associated with poor coordination of the sphincter and detrusor and often the detrusor contracts against a closed sphincter (DSD).

Answers

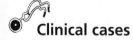

Clinical cases

CASE 5.16 – 'I have leakage and have to go very frequently'

A1: What is the likely differential diagnosis?

- Urine infections.
- Poor catheterization technique.
- General weakness.

A2: What issues in the given history support/refute a particular diagnosis?

In these patients there is usually a failure to store with either a bladder that is overactive or underactive. The management is to define the bladder pressures (high bladder pressures may affect the upper tract leading to obstructive uropathy). Maintain continence by intermittent self-catheterization.

Urinary leak in between catheterizations would indicate either infrequent catheterizations or improper technique (suggesting that the bladder is not being emptied adequately).

Urine infections are also a common cause of urinary leak.

The history of ascending UTIs is in keeping with incomplete emptying of the bladder with some evidence of reflux.

A3: What additional features would you seek to support a particular diagnosis?

Overactive bladder symptoms are generally well correlated with patient symptoms and investigations; however, bladder emptying may not be obtained in history and investigations must be relied on for this.

Spinal cord lesions are commonly associated with DSD: the normal coordinated relaxation of the sphincter to detrusor contraction at the time of voiding is lost. The detrusor contracts against a closed sphincter, thereby generating significant bladder pressures to eventually become transmitted to the kidney. This results in renal damage. The other cause of renal damage as discussed above is high detrusor pressures in filling phase with poor compliance.

A4: What clinical examination would you perform and why?

- Examination of the abdomen to rule out a palpable bladder
- Systemic examination to rule out organomegaly

A5: What investigations would be most helpful and why?

- Urine culture and sensitivity
- Urodynamics: detrusor overactivity of neurogenic origin, often associated with DSD
- Ultrasonography of the renal tract: to assess underlying causes of infection (e.g. stone, large residual volume, damage to upper tracts with renal scarring and dilatation)
- MAG-3 scan: to assess split function of the renal tract
- Video-urodynamics: would confirm detrusor overactivity, DSD, anatomical abnormalities of the urinary tract and reflux of urine into the upper tracts

A6: What treatment options are appropriate?

The urinary symptoms of patients with spinal injuries are commonly managed by intermittent self-catheterization and with anticholinergics. This would ensure that the bladder volumes remain low and reduce the bladder pressure, which is sufficient to retain continence. It also reduces the risk of upper tract damage.

To reduce the bladder pressure it may be necessary to inject Botox into the bladder wall and paralyse the bladder wall and reduce contractions. Another option is to augment the bladder using a patch of detubularized bowel segment onto the bivalved bladder (clam cystoplasty), but this is rarely performed since the introduction of Botox injections.

If incontinence is still a problem, then improvement in the urethral resistance may be achieved by surgically inserting an artificial sphincter which may be regulated to achieve continence.

A surgical procedure is to divide the posterior nerve roots (posterior rhizotomy) and insert a surgical implant in the anterior sacral nerve roots (S2–4). This converts the bladder into an a-reflexic bladder with no sensation. The bladder is drained by stimulating the anterior nerve roots, which may be activated by a subcutaneous transducer.

CASE 5.17 – 'I am unable to pass urine'

A1: What is the likely differential diagnosis?

- MS
- Spinal cord compression or tumour
- Urethral sphincter overactivity
- Pelvic masses and tumours
- Chronic constipation

A2: What issues in the given history support/refute a particular diagnosis?

Multiple sclerosis is three times more common in women and is normally diagnosed between the ages of 20 and 40 years. The common symptoms are fatigue and vision disturbances. Bladder symptoms are usually urgency with neurogenic detrusor overactivity.

A3: What additional features would you seek to support a particular diagnosis?

- UTIs and constipation
- History of ovarian tumours and pelvic masses

A4: What clinical examination would you perform and why?

- Focused examination of the abdomen and pelvis, and DRE
- Neurological examination, including assessment of the motor, sensory and tendon reflexes of lower limbs, and perineal sensation, including bulbocavernosus reflex (BCR), to confirm integrity of the sacral reflex arc. A negative BCR would mean that the patient most probably has a spinal cord lesion, whereas a positive BCR does not rule out a cord lesion.

A5: What investigations would be most helpful and why?

- Urine dipstick and microscopy
- Ultrasonography of abdomen and pelvis
- MRI of spinal cord and cauda equina

A6: What treatment options are appropriate?

Referral to a neurologist is appropriate and the immediate treatment consists of relieving the urinary retention. The long-term outcome depends on progression of the MS.

CASE 5.18 – 'I have recurrent infections'

A1: What is the likely differential diagnosis?

Patients with paraplegia have a tendency to develop urinary tract calculi.

The differential diagnosis is likely to be incomplete emptying of the bladder and re-infection through the use of the poor intermittent self-catheterization technique.

A2: What issues in the given history support/refute a particular diagnosis?

Reflux is notable.

A3: What additional features would you seek to support a particular diagnosis?

Overactive bladder symptoms are in keeping with urgency frequency and urgency incontinence. Urine infections are associated with dysuria and haematuria.

A4: What clinical examination would you perform and why?

- Examination of the abdomen to rule out a palpable bladder
- Systemic examination to rule out organomegaly

A5: What investigations would be most helpful and why?

- Urine culture and sensitivity
- Imaging of the renal tract to rule out stones and increased residual of urine

A6: What treatment options are appropriate?

Improve bladder emptying and treat urinary stone disease. Long-term antibiotics may be helpful but may also foster antibiotic resistance.

REVISION PANEL

- Neuropathic bladder is often due to either detrusor overactivity or underactivity with or without sphincteric overactivity or loss. It may also be classified according to the neurological level: sacral, suprasacral, peripheral and suprapontine.
- The management is often symptomatic to treat urgency and bladder emptying. Failure to store may need medication like anticholinergics and beta-adrenergics.
- Failure to empty may need intermittent self-catheterization and upper tract surveillance to ensure that there is no kidney damage related to high bladder pressure.
- Failure to void is a common symptom in patients with neurological conditions.
- This is managed by stimulated voiding (abdominal pressure, e.g. Crede manoeuvre), intermittent clean self-catheterization, long-term suprapubic or urethral catheters.
- Urinary retention may be one of the early symptoms of a neurological condition (e.g. MS).
- Idiopathic urinary retention in young women is now well defined and may occur due to increased activity in the sphincter mechanism.
- Recurrent infections are common in patients with neurogenic bladder dysfunction. This may be due to incomplete emptying and also associated with abnormality of the urinary tract or stone formation.
- The management is often symptomatic to treat urgency and bladder emptying and infections. Failure to void may need intermittent self/carer catheterization or long-term catheter.
- Long-term catheters may be associated with urinary infections. Intravesical Botox injections may assist in reducing bladder-related complications.

UPPER TRACT OBSTRUCTION AND RENAL MASS

Questions

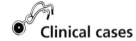
Clinical cases

For each of the clinical case scenarios given

> **Q1:** What is the likely differential diagnosis?
> **Q2:** What issues in the given history support/refute a particular diagnosis?
> **Q3:** What additional features would you seek to support a particular diagnosis?
> **Q4:** What clinical examination would you perform and why?
> **Q5:** What investigations would be most helpful and why?
> **Q6:** What treatment options are appropriate?

CASE 5.19 – 'I have pain in my loin when I have a drink'

A 25-year-old woman presents to her GP with significant pain in her loin and nausea and vomiting after a night out with her friends. She has had a similar episode before and has had an episode of urinary infection in the past.

CASE 5.20 – A 57-year-old man with advanced malignancy has bilateral hydronephrosis

A 57-year-old man presents with a recurrent colorectal tumour with advanced metastatic disease and a mass in the pelvis. He is unwell with weight loss, loss of appetite and nausea. Ultrasonography reveals bilateral hydronephrosis and a mass in the pelvis.

CASE 5.21 – 'I have lost weight and have a loss of appetite and a lump in my belly'

A 63-year-old man presents with a rapidly painful swelling of his left testicle, a mass in his abdomen and haematuria. He has had a loss of appetite and lost a stone (about 7 kg) in weight over the last 3 months. He has also been feeling quite tired.

OSCE Counselling case

OSCE COUNSELLING CASE 5.8 – 'How do I counsel a patient for a nephrostomy?'

A 23-year-old woman with fever and confusion and who is systemically unwell undergoes ultrasonography to reveal a right-sided hydronephrosis. There is a stone seen in the renal pelvis. She has previously had significant UTIs. She has been started on antibiotics but she has not improved.

Q1: What would you need to discuss with her before consent for a nephrostomy?

Key concepts

- Upper urinary tract obstruction
- Acute or chronic obstruction

Hydronephrosis is a descriptive term associated with a pathological dilatation of the renal pelvis and calyces. Dilatation may be the result of an obstruction to the urinary tract, which may be unilateral or bilateral, acute or chronic, complete or incomplete.

A PUJ abnormality is caused by a short stenotic segment at the level of the PUJ. In the normal kidney, pacemakers in the minor calyces initiate a contraction wave, which passes down to the lower ureter. The normal spiral muscle of the PUJ and the ureter may be replaced by a localized longitudinal segment which does not allow coordinated proximal contractions to reach the lower ureter. This may also be caused by an abnormal lower-pole vessel crossing the proximal ureter.

Non-obstructive dilatation of the renal pelvis may be vesicoureteric reflux, dysplasia or problems in the developmental anatomy of the urinary tract.

The most common causes of upper urinary tract obstruction are urinary stone disease, sloughed renal papilla, blood clot, acute retroperitoneal pathology and accidental ligation of the ureter.

Bilateral obstruction of the upper tracts is a result of a lower urinary tract obstruction, with backpressure onto both kidneys (e.g. prostatic obstruction or obstruction to both the ureters caused by a retroperitoneal pathology). Recovery of the obstruction after its relief is initially by the recovery of the tubular function and is followed by a much slower glomerular recovery.

RENAL MASSES

The most common presentation is haematuria and loin pain. An increasing number are being diagnosed incidentally with increasing use of ultrasonography for diagnosis. Thirty per cent note a mass in the abdomen or have symptoms of metastatic disease with weight loss and loss of appetite. The classic triad of 'haematuria, pain and a loin mass' is rare and occurs in about 10 per cent of cases. Involvement of the renal vein and obstruction of the left testicular vein results in presentation with an acute varicocoele.

Renal tumours may mimic a range of conditions as a result of the paraneoplastic syndromes caused by ectopic hormone secretion or mediated by interleukin-6 (common syndromes associated with renal tumours are anaemia, polycythaemia, hypertension, Cushing's syndrome, reversible hepatic dysfunction [Stauffer's syndrome] and pyrexia with night sweats).

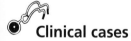

Answers

Clinical cases

CASE 5.19 – 'I have pain in my loin when I have a drink'

A1: What is the likely differential diagnosis?

Upper ureteric obstruction may be the result of the following:

- PUJ obstruction
- Ureteric stone
- Upper ureteric tumour
- Sloughed-off renal papilla
- Ureteric strictures (infective, e.g. tuberculous/iatrogenic/radiation induced or due to malignancy)
- Renal pelvis dilatation without obstruction that may be the result of reflux of urine into the renal pelvis from the bladder or of a dilated but non-obstructed renal pelvis

A2: What issues in the given history support/refute a particular diagnosis?

Pelviureteric junction obstruction is due to an obstruction from the renal pelvis and the proximal ureter. This may present in both adults and children with loin pain, hydronephrosis, recurrent urine infections or stone formation. The diagnosis is suspected when pain is brought on by forced diuresis (e.g. alcohol intake).

A3: What additional features would you seek to support a particular diagnosis?

Urinary stone disease with ureteric calculi may be the cause of unilateral kidney obstruction and often presents with renal colic associated or without microscopic haematuria.

Urinary tract obstruction may be due to renal papillary necrosis (e.g. sloughed-off renal papilla associated with diabetics and analgesia abuse).

The upper ureteric tumour was associated with phenacetin-containing analgesic abuse and smoking (phenacetin has consequently been discontinued in the United Kingdom). It is more common in males and appears to peak in the seventh decade. These tumours are more common in the distal third of the ureter and are commonly associated with synchronous bladder tumours.

A4: What clinical examination would you perform and why?

The loin mass may be palpable.

A5: What investigations would be most helpful and why?

- IVU: chronic obstruction is often identified and information about the anatomy is usually obtained. This usually requires a reasonable renal function and glomerular filtration rate (GFR), and is usually not helpful if the creatinine is >200 mmol/L.
- Ultrasonography: this is non-invasive and a useful screening tool; it identifies hydronephrosis, and the renal cortical thickness gives a rough assessment of the chronicity of the condition and the possibility of recovery of function.
- Isotope diuresis renography: radioactive tracers are tagged to molecules that are effectively cleared by the first pass through the kidney through a combination of partial filtration and active tubular secretion. Technetium-99m (^{99m}Tc)-labelled mercaptoacetyl triglycine (MAG-3) is commonly used

intravenously, and the renal handling of the radioactive tracer is monitored with gamma scanners over the abdomen and plotted against time. A persistent accumulation of the tracer in the kidney not eliminated by a diuretic is consistent with obstruction. A slow elimination caused by urinary stasis in a dilated renal pelvis responds to an increased urinary flow with a rapid washout of the tracer following the diuretic.

A6: What treatment options are appropriate?

It is important to note that dilatation does not necessarily mean obstruction.
The following questions are helpful in planning the treatment:

- Is the dilatation the result of an active obstruction or is it a non-obstructive dilatation?
- Is the function of the kidney in obstructed kidneys sufficient to justify correction? A nephrectomy is more appropriate in poorly functioning kidneys.

Defining the anatomical level of the obstruction

It is important to define obstruction before performing an operation for relief of the obstruction. An operation is commonly performed to correct obstruction when there is a deterioration of renal function of the affected renal unit (<40 per cent of the split function), symptoms of pain, haematuria, and the development of complications from the obstruction.

A PUJ obstruction is a short stenotic segment that may be incised, dilated or excised and re-anastomosed (Anderson-Hynes pyeloplasty).

CASE 5.20 – A 57-year-old man with advanced malignancy has bilateral hydronephrosis

A1: What is the likely differential diagnosis?

- Chronic urinary retention with high bladder pressures may cause bilateral hydronephrosis.
- Bilateral hydronephrosis may be the result of an obstruction to the prostate or bladder neck or to both ureters.

A2: What issues in the given history support/refute a particular diagnosis?

Chronic urinary retention with a palpable bladder may point towards an infra-vesical obstruction leading to bilateral hydronephrosis.

Advanced malignancy is associated with retroperitoneal pathology and may involve both the ureters, causing bilateral hydronephrosis.

A3: What additional features would you seek to support a particular diagnosis?

Symptoms of bladder outflow obstruction.
Duration of symptoms may be useful in estimating loss of renal function.
Prognosis from the advanced malignancy and treatment options is available, and the patient's choice of treatment needs to be ascertained.

A4: What clinical examination would you perform and why?

Is the bladder palpable? Is there a palpable mass in the abdomen or pelvis on pelvic examination?

A5: What investigations would be most helpful and why?

- Renal function tests are useful.

- Dilatation of the renal tract is often identified with an ultrasound scan. The thickness of the renal cortex often allows interpretation of the duration of the obstruction and reversible nature of obstruction. A thin renal cortex often implies long-standing disease with irreversible renal damage.
- CT is used to assess retroperitoneum and pelvic masses or to stage a neoplastic disease.

A6: What treatment options are appropriate?

Chronic urinary retention is managed by prompt urinary catheterization and drainage of the bladder. Renal damage related to high-pressure chronic retention needs to be assessed and monitored to treat electrolyte abnormality appropriately.

Stenting the ureters to remove obstructions is commonly done anterograde after emergency placement of nephrostomies either into both kidneys or into the better-functioning kidney.

The decision to treat ureters obstructed by malignancy must be discussed openly with the patient because this would prolong life, with the progression of metastatic disease and all the symptoms from that. If a good quality of life can be obtained from treatment of the obstructed kidneys, it may be considered together with the patient, oncologist and palliative consultant.

CASE 5.21 – 'I have lost weight and have a loss of appetite and a lump in my belly'

A1: What is the likely differential diagnosis?

Renal masses with weight loss and loss of appetite may be caused by the following:

- Renal tumour
- Infective granulomatous changes with XGPN
- Paraneoplastic syndromes that may mimic a whole range of conditions
- A renal cyst that is infected or haemorrhage in a renal cyst which may present with pain and a mass

A2: What issues in the given history support/refute a particular diagnosis?

Renal tumours have a unique propensity to spread via the renal vein, and the tumour thrombus may also involve the inferior vena cava or even up to the right atrium. Renal vein involvement on the left side may impair drainage of the testicular vein that may result in a new-onset varicocoele in an adult.

A renal mass with haematuria is commonly associated with an underlying renal tumour.

A3: What additional features would you seek to support a particular diagnosis?

History of stone disease with recurrent infections is common with renal mass that is associated with infection and results in a XGPN.

A4: What clinical examination would you perform and why?

Examination of the renal mass and test for anaemia should be performed.

A5: What investigations would be most helpful and why?

Contrast CT of chest and abdomen and pelvis would assist in staging of the renal tumour and assessment of the renal vein and inferior vena cava. Distant metastasis and lymph node involvement may also be obtained from this.

Urine cytology and urine culture would help to rule out infection.

In paraneoplastic syndromes associated with renal cancers, polycythaemia or anaemia may occur. Hypercalcaemia may be associated with a para-neoplastic process in renal cancer.

Liver function tests would show hepatic dysfunction that is reversible after nephrectomy which is described as 'Stauffer's syndrome'.

Renal tumours have been known to be a cause for pyrexia, possibly due to IL-6 production by the tumour.

A6: What treatment options are appropriate?

A radical nephrectomy is the recommended treatment with a curative intent.

Metastatic disease generally has a poor prognosis. The primary tumour should be removed if it is causing symptoms and the patient is fit. Debulking nephrectomy in metastatic disease may be followed by systemic immunotherapy with tyrosine kinase inhibitors to improve survival.

ⅲ OSCE Counselling case

OSCE COUNSELLING CASE 5.8 – 'How do I counsel a patient for a nephrostomy?'

Nephrostomy is to insert a tube to drain the kidney. This is often done under screening percutaneously using either an image intensifier or ultrasound scan. The indications are to drain a renal unit that is obstructed or pus from an obstructed renal system.

Nephrostomy is associated with 1 per cent mortality and with loss of renal unit as a result of bleeding.

Percutaneous nephrostomy is usually performed by the radiologist or a urologist often using an image intensifier or ultrasound screening.

Obstructed renal units lose function often over 6 weeks. However, an infected obstructed renal unit deteriorates function extremely rapidly often within a few hours. The drainage of pus should be sent for culture and sensitivity and appropriate antibiotics started as soon as possible.

REVISION PANEL

- Unilateral hydronephrosis may be due to obstruction. The common causes are acute obstruction related to ureteric stones, clots or renal papillary necrosis. The presentation is with severe loin pain with or without haematuria.
- Chronic unilateral obstruction may be due to chronic obstruction of the renal collecting system that may be related to anatomical obstruction of the ureter. This may be due to extrinsic compression of the ureter from pelvic malignancy or recurrence.
- Congenital abnormality of the junction between the renal pelvis and proximal ureter may lead to PUJ that may present at any time as an adult or child. The symptoms are related to loin pain, haematuria, stone formation or urine infections.
- Dilatation of the tract may lead to hydronephrosis or hydroureter. Obstruction is defined by assessing the drainage of the radioactive tracer and delay in an obstructed system using a MAG-3 scan.
- The treatment is to define the cause of the obstruction, identify split function of the kidney and relieve the obstruction. If, however, the function of the kidney is significantly lost, this may result in a nephrectomy.
- Bilateral hydronephrosis may be due to bilateral ureteric obstructions either from stones, extrinsic compression by stricture, pelvic mass or retroperitoneal structures. The most common cause however is infravesical obstruction due to chronic urinary retention.
- The presence of a palpable bladder or significant residual volume is suggestive of chronic urinary retention that may require prompt bladder drainage and monitoring to treat probable reversible renal damage related to obstruction.
- Bilateral ureteric obstruction may be due to infiltration of the ureteric orifices or ureters in the retroperitoneum. Infiltration of the trigone and ureteric orifices may be due to bladder or prostate neoplasm. This is often indicative of advanced disease.
- Ureteric obstruction may be noted in retroperitoneal disease following radiation, following surgery and scarring or due to extensive malignancy. The diagnosis of the cause of the obstruction, residual function of the kidneys and split renal function may assist in management.
- Obstruction to the renal tract is often treated with drainage either using a nephrostomy or by ureteric stent insertion done either antegrade from the nephrostomy tract or retrograde from the bladder. This is followed by treatment of the cause of obstruction if possible.
- Renal tumours may present with a triad of renal mass, haematuria and loin pain. This triad of symptoms is only infrequently noted and often renal tumours are identified incidentally by ultrasound or CT imaging for other indications.
- Renal tumours may involve a tumour thrombus that spreads into the renal vein and may also progress into the IVC and even the right atrium. New-onset varicocoele from obstruction of gonadal vein from thrombus may be an indication of a renal tumour and urgent ultrasound scan of the renal tract as well as the varicocoele is recommended.
- Renal tumours are often treated by nephrectomy. The presence of metastasis does not preclude surgery. Salvage nephrectomy following by immunotherapy or anti-angiogenesis medication may improve survival.

SCROTAL PAIN, TESTICULAR LUMPS

Questions

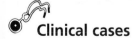

Clinical cases

For each of the clinical case scenarios given

> **Q1:** What is the likely differential diagnosis?
> **Q2:** What issues in the given history support/refute a particular diagnosis?
> **Q3:** What additional features would you seek to support a particular diagnosis?
> **Q4:** What clinical examination would you perform and why?
> **Q5:** What investigations would be most helpful and why?
> **Q6:** What treatment options are appropriate?

CASE 5.22 – 'I have noticed a lump in my scrotum. Have I got cancer?'

A 24-year-old man presents with a painless lump in his scrotum that he noticed in the shower. He is fit and well and is a non-smoker.

CASE 5.23 – A 22-year-old man presents with painful swelling of his scrotum

A 22-year-old man presents with a painful lump in his scrotum. He has mild dysuria and has had treatment for chlamydial urethritis in the past.

CASE 5.24 – 'My son is complaining of a painful scrotum and is not able to walk'

A parent's son is 9 years old and has woken up with a painful scrotum and is unable to walk; the scrotum is red and tender. He has never had any problems before.

🔑 Key concepts

Testicular cancer is common in young men (20 to 45 years). It is now one of the most curable cancers. Teratomas usually occur at a younger age than seminomas (20 to 35 versus 35 to 45 years). It is associated with undescended testis and contralateral testicular tumour. Testicular tumours are associated with HIV infection.

Germ cell tumours are classified as seminomatous or non-seminomatous (Table 5.2). The latter include teratomas.

There are two types of torsion: that inside the tunica vaginalis (intravaginal, most common) and that outside (extravaginal). Testicular torsion is an emergency because irreversible ischaemic damage occurs within 4 hours.

In patients who are prone to an intravaginal torsion in the testis, the space between the layers of the tunica vaginalis extends high up into the spermatic cord. This creates an abnormally mobile testis that hangs freely within the space of the tunica (a 'bell-clapper deformity'), allowing the testis to twist in the axis of the cord.

Torsion is recognized by sudden onset of pain and swelling of the testicle. There is often a history of previous severe self-limiting scrotal pain. Dysuria and bladder symptoms are absent. It is worth noting that 90 per cent of adolescents presenting with severe scrotal pain and swelling have a torsion.

Epididymo-orchitis occurs in all age groups and must be differentiated from testicular torsion and testicular tumour. The typical presentation is a gradual onset of testicular pain and swelling associated with scrotal redness and a hydrocoele. In men under 40 years the most common causative organisms are *Chlamydia* spp., gonococci and coliforms. Coliforms and other Gram-negative organisms are more common in those aged over 40 years. The aetiology in children is commonly abacterial (often viral, i.e. mumps).

Table 5.2 Germ-Cell and Non-Germ-Cell Tumours

Germ-Cell Tumours	Non-Germ-Cell Tumours (Relatively Rare)
Seminoma	Leydig cell tumours
Teratoma	Sertoli cell tumours
Yolk sac tumour	Granulosa cell tumours
Trophoblastic tumour (choriocarcinoma)	Mixed

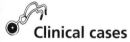

Answers

Clinical cases

CASE 5.22 – 'I have noticed a lump in my scrotum. Have I got cancer?'

A1: What is the likely differential diagnosis?

Testicular lumps

- Testicular cancer
- Epididymal cyst
- Hydrocoele
- Hernia
- Varicocoele

A2: What issues in the given history support/refute a particular diagnosis?

Testicular tumours occur in young adults and are often painless.

A3: What additional features would you seek to support a particular diagnosis?

- History of an undescended testis is an important risk factor.
- Sperm granulomas with a painful lump in the cord may be present after a vasectomy.
- Hydrocoele is a globular swelling in the scrotum that is not painful.
- A cough impulse is commonly present with a hernia.
- Metastatic disease from testicular cancer may present with shortness of breath, back pain and nipple tenderness.

A4: What clinical examination would you perform and why?

- Physical examination to reveal supraclavicular lymph nodes, chest signs, hepatomegaly, abdominal mass and lower limb oedema
- Testicular examination to reveal a hard mass in the testis
- Examination of hydrocoele that is fluctuant and transilluminates
- Exclusion of inguinoscrotal hernia with the ability to get above the mass at the level of the spermatic cord

A5: What investigations would be most helpful and why?

- Ultrasonography: distinguishes solid and fluid-filled scrotal lesions
- Testicular tumour markers:
  - β-Human chorionic gonadotropin (β-hCG): 40 per cent of teratomas and 15 per cent of seminomas
  - Lactate dehydrogenase (LDH): 10 to 20 per cent of seminomas
  - α-Fetoprotein (AFP): 50 to 70 per cent of teratomas and yolk sac tumours
- Abdominal and chest contrast CT for staging for para-aortic lymphadenopathy and soft tissue metastasis

A6: What treatment options are appropriate?

The primary treatment of all testicular tumours is a radical orchidectomy through a groin incision. Further treatment depends on the staging CT and tumour markers. Systemic disease is commonly treated with combination chemotherapy or radiotherapy.

Residual lymph nodal disease after chemotherapy may be resected by a retroperitoneal lymph node dissection.

CASE 5.23 – **A 22-year-old man presents with painful swelling of his scrotum**

A1: What is the likely differential diagnosis?

- Epididymo-orchitis
- Testicular torsion
- Testicular tumour with a bleed
- Strangulated hernia

A2: What issues in the given history support/refute a particular diagnosis?

A history of previous urethritis may suggest an infective process; an epididymo-orchitis is commonly associated with dysuria and bladder symptoms. The onset of symptoms is more gradual and associated with scrotal redness and may have a moderate hydrocoele.

A3: What additional features would you seek to support a particular diagnosis?

- Acute testicular torsion is common in younger patients with sudden onset of symptoms. In addition pain is more prominent than tenderness, whereas in epididymo-orchitis tenderness is the main feature.
- A history of sexual activity and promiscuity is important to consider. Previous sexually transmitted infections (STIs) and contact tracing are an important aspect of the management.
- A strangulated inguinoscrotal hernia is commonly associated with nausea and vomiting. Patients are often systemically unwell.

A4: What clinical examination would you perform and why?

Scrotal examination would be useful to perform. Epididymo-orchitis is associated with a tender swelling of the epididymis. It has a vertical lie and the epididymis is posterior. It may be associated with a small hydrocoele.

Testicular tumour is a hard, non-tender mass involving part or the whole of the testis.

A5: What investigations would be most helpful and why?

- Urine microscopy and culture: isolate organism
- Urethral swab for *Chlamydia* spp.
- Ultrasonography of scrotum: differentiates solid and cystic masses
- Colour Doppler study: not commonly done but useful to assess vascularity of the testis

A6: What treatment options are appropriate?

In men aged under 40 years doxycycline or a quinolone for 10 days is appropriate. If gonococci are suspected a single intramuscular dose of ceftriaxone should be added to doxycycline.

In men aged over 40 years a fluoroquinolone for 10 days may be sufficient.

CASE 5.24 – 'My son is complaining of a painful scrotum and is not able to walk'

A1: What is the likely differential diagnosis?

- Testicular torsion
- Torsion of a testicular appendage
- Epididymo-orchitis
- Idiopathic scrotal oedema

A2: What issues in the given history support/refute a particular diagnosis?

Torsion of the testicle on the spermatic cord is common around puberty. The symptoms are sudden in onset with pain and nausea and vomiting. There may be local redness and the testis may be lying higher in the root of the scrotum.

A3: What additional features would you seek to support a particular diagnosis?

A history of sharp intermittent pains that are self-limiting may be present and signify previous intermittent torsions that have resolved.

A4: What clinical examination would you perform and why?

The testis may be horizontal or retracted up to the root of the scrotum. The testis is usually swollen and exquisitely tender. A cremasteric reflex is often absent and may be a useful indicator.

A5: What investigations would be most helpful and why?

Ultrasound and colour Doppler assessment are operator dependent and may delay prompt surgical intervention; they are considered only if the diagnosis is doubtful.

A6: What treatment options are appropriate?

A manual de-torsion may be attempted but this must not delay an urgent exploration of the testicle. The testis is examined for signs of ischaemia; if normal it is repositioned and fixed to the tunica vaginalis with non-absorbable, non-reactive sutures. If nonviable testis is present despite attempts to improve vascularization and oxygenation (warm saline packs around testes, increased oxygenation of patient and detorsion), this may result in an orchiectomy of the necrotic testis.

REVISION PANEL

- A painless testicular lump is often indicative of testicular tumour and regular self-examination of testes is usually recommended as a screening tool.
- Testicular tumours are treated by radical orchidectomy followed by additional treatment depending on the grade and stage of disease.
- Serum tumour markers are available to identify the tumour and for monitoring treatment if elevated.
- Advanced germ cell tumours may present with intra-abdominal lymphadenopathy or metastatic disease. The primary tumour may often be impalpable as a 'burned out' primary testicular tumour requiring an ultrasound scan to identify this.
- Unilateral painful swelling of the testes may be related to epididymo-orchitis.
- Voiding symptoms or indwelling foreign bodies like urethral catheter may be associated with related epididymo-orchitis coliform infection.
- Urethral discharge or history of STI may be related to a chlamydial epididymo-orchitis.
- Epididymo-orchitis may result in severe pain and often scrotal abscess.
- Testicular torsion is a clinical diagnosis and prompt scrotal exploration is indicated to avoid loss of the testis.
- The clinical diagnosis is based on unilateral testicular pain that is of sudden onset associated with clinical examination of an abnormal lie of the testis that is often higher than the other testis in the absence of any inflammatory features.
- Scrotal exploration within 6 to 8 hours usually leads to salvage of a viable testis.
- Unilateral orchidectomy of the necrotic testes may become necessary if there has been a delayed diagnosis.

ERECTILE DYSFUNCTION/INFERTILITY

Questions

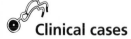 **Clinical cases**

For each of the clinical case scenarios given

> **Q1:** What is the likely differential diagnosis?
> **Q2:** What issues in the given history support/refute a particular diagnosis?
> **Q3:** What additional features would you seek to support a particular diagnosis?
> **Q4:** What clinical examination would you perform and why?
> **Q5:** What investigations would be most helpful and why?
> **Q6:** What treatment options are appropriate?

CASE 5.25 – 'I am unable to have erections'

A 45-year-old man newly diagnosed with diabetes presents with difficulty having erections for the last 6 months. He does not have adequately rigid erections and is unable to maintain them.

CASE 5.26 – 'We have been trying for a child for 3 years'

A couple have had unprotected intercourse for 3 years and have not conceived. He had repair of an undescended testicle as a child.

CASE 5.27 – 'I have an ulcer on my penis'

A 78-year-old man has had a foul-smelling discharge from his foreskin for several months and on clinical examination has a fungating mass on the end of his penis.

OSCE Counselling case

OSCE COUNSELLING CASE 5.9 – **Counsel a 35-year-old patient for a vasectomy**

A 35-year-old man has requested a vasectomy; he and his partner have three children, have completed their family and would like a permanent sterilization.

Key concepts

Erectile dysfunction is the inability to obtain a satisfactory erection for sexual intercourse.

The male factors of infertility or subfertility are the following: men with one or both undescended testicles regardless of the age at orchidopexy, mumps or orchitis after puberty and substance abuse.

Penile carcinoma is uncommon but occurs in elderly men. The premalignant conditions associated with penile cancers appear as chronic, painless, red or pale patches and include leukoplakia and erythroplasia of Queyrat.

Infections with human papilloma virus (HPV)-16, -18 and -21 are important and associated with cervical cancer in the partner. Circumcision as a neonate may confer some protection against penile cancer, and this may be related to the chronic irritation from the smegma and balanitis in men with poor hygiene.

The most common cancer is a squamous carcinoma which may be preceded by carcinoma in situ of the glans or the foreskin. Metastasis is to the inguinal lymph nodes and then to the pelvic lymph nodes. Blood-borne metastasis to the lungs and liver is rare.

The common presentation is a hard painless lump or a malignant ulcer on the penis.

Vasectomy is a permanent form of sterilization. There are several techniques that are used. The principle involves isolating the vas deferens, delivering it through a small skin incision and dividing a portion of it.

Answers

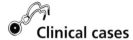

Clinical cases

CASE 5.25 – 'I am unable to have erections'

A1: What is the likely differential diagnosis?

Psychogenic erectile dysfunction is the most common cause and is associated with stress, performance anxiety and previous sexual relationship problems.

Organic erectile dysfunction may also occur as a result of disruption of nerve conduction caused by neurological processes such as Parkinson's disease, stroke, head trauma and nerve disruption, as in a radical prostatectomy.

Arterial occlusive disease of the pudendal cavernous helicine arteries can reduce arterial inflow to the sinusoids. Common risk factors include hypertension, hyperlipidaemia, cigarette smoking and diabetes.

Causes are also drug induced and due to hypogonadism (pituitary or gonadal).

A2: What issues in the given history support/refute a particular diagnosis?

Diabetes is a common cause of erectile dysfunction.

A3: What additional features would you seek to support a particular diagnosis?

Erectile dysfunction that is gradual and insidious in onset is more likely to be organic. It is often associated with loss of spontaneous or early morning erections.

On the contrary, erectile dysfunction related to periods of stress (e.g. marital, financial and psychological stress) is commonly sudden in onset, and spontaneous erections are often preserved.

Drug-induced erectile dysfunction is common with centrally acting antihypertensives, antipsychotics and antidepressants.

Chronic alcoholism and smoking are known to affect erection adversely.

A4: What clinical examination would you perform and why?

Examination of the breasts, hair distribution, testes and thyroid would be conducted to detect an endocrine abnormality.

Femoral and foot pulses would be checked for vascular insufficiency.

Genital and perineal sensation would be examined for neurological deficit and penile abnormalities.

Clinical syndromes such as Klinefelter's syndrome are associated with a typical appearance.

A5: What investigations would be most helpful and why?

- Hormonal evaluation: serum prolactin, luteinizing hormone (LH), follicle-stimulating hormone (FSH) and testosterone (if evidence of low testosterone on clinical examination), thyroid hormones, liver and renal function tests
- Serum glucose: diabetes

Tests that are rarely performed:

- Duplex ultrasonography: measures penile blood flow velocity
- Cavernosography: identifies a venous leak, but is fraught with false positives and is rarely performed

- Nocturnal tumescence testing: to access sleep-related erection; useful in differentiating psychogenic erectile dysfunction (where nocturnal erections are preserved) from the organic erectile dysfunction (nocturnal erections are lost); performed using a Rigiscan device

A6: What treatment options are appropriate?

- General principles include cessation of smoking, reduction of alcohol intake, consumption of a healthy diet and participation in exercise. Remove precipitating factors such as drugs, long-distance cycling.
- If a psychological component is present, refer to a psychosexual counsellor.
- Treatment depends on patient suitability and preference.
- Oral medications include phospodiesterase inhibitors (sildenafil, vardenafil, tadalafil). PDE5 inhibitors are contraindicated if the patient is on any form of nitrate therapy (e.g. GTN spray or long-acting nitrates).
- Major side effects are headaches, flushing and dyspepsia; use caution with cardiac patients on nitrates (associated with fatal hypotension and arrhythmia).
- Sublingual apomorphine acts on the central dopaminergic receptors and induces erections. The side effects include nausea and vomiting.
- A vacuum device can be placed over the penis and a pump produces a vacuum; a constricting ring is placed on the base of the penis to maintain the rigidity after the penis is engorged by the negative pressure. A retained ejaculate and numbness of the penis are some of the side effects.
- Intracavernosal injections: papaverine and alprostadil are used and this is one of the most effective and reliable second-line therapies for erectile dysfunction. There is a risk of persistent erection lasting more than 4 hours (priapism) that requires urgent decompression.
- Penile prosthesis is implanted into the corpora and replaces the normal erectile tissue; the prosthesis may be solid (rigid or semirigid) and is malleable. The most common prosthesis is the inflatable device with a reservoir and pump and inflatable rods that are implanted into the corpora.

CASE 5.26 – 'We have been trying for a child for 3 years'

A1: What is the likely differential diagnosis?

Male causes of primary infertility
- Hypothalamic causes: hypogonadotrophic hypogonadism: Kallmann's syndrome
- Pituitary causes: surgery, irradiation, infarction, tumours, infections
- Hormonal excess: anabolic steroids, congenital adrenal hyperplasia, excess oestrogens and prolactinomas
- Chromosomal: Klinefelter's syndrome (XXY)
- Systemic diseases: uraemia, liver failure
- Testicular causes: orchitis (postpubertal), undescended testes, trauma, infections, varicocoele
- Cystic fibrosis: associated with bilateral vasal agenesis

A2: What issues in the given history support/refute a particular diagnosis?

History of an undescended testis as a child is important.

A3: What additional features would you seek to support a particular diagnosis?

- Duration of infertility and prior pregnancies; details of sexual history and potency and use of lubricants are important.
- History of previous surgery to the vas or pelvis and infections (e.g. mumps, trauma to testis) are important.
- History of diabetes and drug history and family history of cystic fibrosis are important.

A4: What clinical examination would you perform and why?

- General examination: body hair distribution, gynaecomastia
- Examination of genitalia, size of the testis, thickening of epididymis
- Examination for penile abnormalities (e.g. hypospadias)
- Examination for presence of a vas deferens
- Examine for presence of a varicocoele

A5: What investigations would be most helpful and why?

- Urine: microscopy to rule out infection and to assess for sperm (retrograde ejaculation)
- Semen analysis: oligospermia/azoospermia sperm counts
- Asthenospermia
- Hormonal evaluation: LH, FSH, testosterone and prolactin
- Testicular biopsy: in azoospermia to differentiate between obstructive and non-obstructive forms; reported as a Johnsen's score 0 to 10 and a score >8 would suggest that the sperm is useful for intracytoplasmic sperm injection (ICSI)/in vitro fertilization (IVF)
- In cases of obstructive azoospermia: transrectal ultrasonography to assess the fullness of the seminal vesicles and vasography to identify the level of the block
- Rare tests: postcoital tests/anti-sperm antibodies (in serum, seminal plasma), karyotyping and cystic fibrosis mutation testing

A6: What treatment options are appropriate?

A combined cause is noted in 30 per cent of cases and a purely male factor for infertility is noted in 20 per cent of cases.

- For post-testicular causes: after vasectomy or focal obstruction: the block is identified using a vasography. A vasovasostomy or vasoepididymostomy is performed.
- Testicular causes: varicocoele is a common cause for infertility and this is repaired either by an open technique (ligation of spermatic veins) or by a laparoscopic technique.
- Correction of the hormone abnormalities is attempted.
- Investigation for a prolactinoma and appropriate management is undertaken.

CASE 5.27 – 'I have an ulcer on my penis'

A1: What is the likely differential diagnosis?

- Carcinoma of the penis
- Balanitis xerotica obliterans: white patch involving prepuce and glans and also the meatus
- Leukoplakia: rare condition, common in those with diabetes, white plaque involves meatus
- Condyloma acuminata: viral origin – HPV

A2: What issues in the given history support/refute a particular diagnosis?

Carcinoma of the penis is more common in older patients. It may develop as an ulcer (typical shallow erosion/excavated ulcer with rolled-out edges) or an exophytic lesion. It eventually develops into a fungating mass and has a purulent smell.

Circumcision in the neonate is protective and it is believed that the presence of smegma and poor hygiene are contributory.

A3: What additional features would you seek to support a particular diagnosis?

- The aetiology is linked to HPV-16 and occurs in partners with carcinoma of the cervix (thought to be linked to HPV).

- Smoking is a known risk factor for carcinoma of the penis.
- The metastatic spread of penile carcinoma is to the lymph nodes and then to the distant organs (lungs/liver/bone).
- Carcinoma in situ (Bowen's disease, when it appears in the shaft of the penis, and erythroplasia of Queyrat, when it appears as a red velvety lesion with ulceration on the glans penis) is a precursor for squamous carcinoma of the penis.

A4: What clinical examination would you perform and why?

General examination is needed to assess the nutritional status, hygiene and general well-being of the patient.

The diagnosis is made by clinical examination and in some circumstances a biopsy may be necessary. Assess the ulcer (size, shape, base, edge, site and involvement of the shaft of the penis and bodies of the corpora). Inguinal lymph nodes may be palpable and in 50 per cent of the cases they are enlarged as a result of infection of the ulcer and not as a result of metastatic spread of the cancer.

A5: What investigations would be most helpful and why?

- Culture swab
- Biopsy of the lesion may be necessary in suspicious circumstances
- Primary tumour (corporal involvement): MRI
- Lymph node involvement: CT of groin, pelvis, abdomen and chest
- Bone scan: distant metastases

A6: What treatment options are appropriate?

Prognosis depends on the following:

- Histological classification (Broder's grade 1 to 3 with 5-year survival rate of 80 per cent in grade 1 and of 30 per cent in grade 3)
- Depth of invasion
- Pattern of growth (superficial spreading, vertical growing, verrucous and multicentric)
- Vascular invasion

Carcinoma in situ may be treated with penis-conserving treatment: topical chemotherapy (e.g. 5-fluorouracil) or glansectomy with resurfacing.

The primary lesion of carcinoma of the penis is treated by excision. Penis-conserving surgery may be performed for lesions involving only the glans. A tumour that involves the corpus spongiosus or cavernosus (T2), or the urethra and prostate (T3), is treated by excision of the lesion with a margin (partial or total penectomy).

A 4-week course of antibiotics often allows differentiation of the lymph nodes with cancer from the ones that are enlarged as a result of infection.

If no palpable nodes are present a prophylactic lymph node dissection of superficial inguinal lymph nodes, and if the frozen section is positive an ipsilateral deep inguinal and pelvic node dissection, is performed in high-grade G3 tumour and high-stage T2–4 disease.

In low-grade G1–2 tumour and T1 disease with no lymph nodes a protocol for surveillance is acceptable, but with a 2-month follow-up.

The presence of nodes after the antibiotic course would require a full dissection of ipsilateral lymph nodes (superficial/deep inguinal/pelvic) and contralateral superficial lymph nodes.

A positive pelvic lymph node is associated with a very poor prognosis: 5-year survival rate of 10 per cent. Chemotherapy is considered for large lymph nodal metastasis and pelvic nodal metastasis.

ĭĭ OSCE Counselling case

OSCE COUNSELLING CASE 5.9 – **Counsel a 35-year-old patient for a vasectomy**

Vasectomy is a permanent form of sterilization and a decision needs to be made by both partners.

The contraindications for vasectomy are mainly relative: clotting abnormalities, local infections and skin abnormalities. Appropriate counselling of couples with a pregnant partner who request a vasectomy is necessary to take into account the risk of stillbirth or perinatal mortality.

A reversal of vasectomy is not as successful (success depends on time between vasectomy and reversal). Microsurgical techniques have a success rate of 60 to 80 per cent, with much lower paternity rates.

Vasectomy is not foolproof. Success is confirmed by negative semen analysis in the third and fourth months after vasectomy. Late recanalization after a negative semen analysis may occur up to 15 years after the procedure in 1:2000.

Persistence of semen in the tract will account for positive semen analysis; a guarded clearance may be given for patients with non-motile sperm of <10000/mL at least 7 months after the vasectomy.

Technique may be by an open vasectomy or a 'no-scalpel technique' using fine sharp instruments to puncture the skin and deliver the vas for ligature – excising a segment of vas and repositioning the ends of the vas either with or without ligation (open-ended vasectomy).

Complications include the sperm granuloma with a painful nodule on the vas. There is post-vasectomy testicular pain/discomfort in up to 18 per cent of patients (caused by epididymal congestion, often treated by non-steroidal anti-inflammatory drugs and rarely requiring reversal of vasectomy). Local complications of haematoma and wound infection are <5 per cent.

REVISION PANEL

- Erectile dysfunction (ED) is often related to endothelial dysfunction and often precedes other organ failures (e.g. myocardial ischaemia or cerebral ischaemia). The history of ED should often be sought out as this may lead to early correction of risk factors for endothelial dysfunction and may prevent strokes or heart attacks.
- Erectile dysfunction is investigated to rule out diabetes or hypogonadism or if there is a psychological cause for this.
- The treatment is often multidisciplinary and oral PDE5 inhibitors have revolutionized the treatment of ED. PDE5 inhibitors are contraindicated in patients on nitrate therapy. Patients with high-risk cardiovascular stratification (unstable angina, recent myocardial infarction, certain arrhythmias and uncontrolled hypertension) should be advised to withhold sexual activity until the medical condition improves.
- Infertility is one of the presentations for patients with Klinefelter's syndrome (47XXY). This accounts for up to 10 per cent of non-obstructive azoospermia. This was originally described as having a triad of gynaecomastia, hypergonadotrophic hypogonadism and infertility. It is often presented with delayed puberty in men with a tall stature, narrow shoulders and shorter torso. Clinical examination often reveals small-volume testes.
- Infertility may be defined on the basis of sperm counts with oligospermia or azoospermia (which may be obstructive or non-obstructive).
- Obstructive azoospermia is associated with a normal testicular biopsy. Non-obstructive azoospermia is often associated with maturation arrest.
- Sperm retrieval and assisted reproduction techniques are commonly used to treat infertility.
- Penile growths are usually squamous cell cancers of the penis.
- This is managed by biopsy and radical excision of the penile lesion.
- Redness and ulceration on the penis need to be examined and biopsied to rule out underlying malignancy.

ACKNOWLEDGEMENT

The contribution of Alan Doherty to this chapter in the first edition is gratefully acknowledged.

Index